FROM
FATIGUED
TO
FANTASTIC!

FROM FATIGUED TO FANTASTIC!

A MANUAL FOR MOVING BEYOND CHRONIC FATIGUE AND FIBROMYALGIA

Jacob Teitelbaum, MD

DEVA PRESS
139 Old Solomons Island Road
Annapolis, Maryland 21401

IMPORTANT NOTICE—DISCLAIMER

This book is written as a general guide for people with Chronic Fatigue Syndrome and Fibromyalgia and others with severe fatigue and those who are working to help them. For obvious reasons, I cannot assume the legal or medical responsibility for having the contents of this book considered as a prescription for anyone.

To conquer your health problems, you will need assistance from a knowledgeable and interested physician or other licensed health care professional. All medical treatments, especially new ones, carry potentially significant medical risks—both known and unforeseen. Accordingly, you and those who work with you must take full responsibility for the uses made of this book. We will be happy to refund the purchase price to anyone who does not accept these conditions.

From Fatigued to Fantastic!
A Manual for Moving Beyond Chronic Fatigue Syndrome and Fibromyalgia
by Jacob Teitelbaum, M.D.

©1995 by Jacob Teitelbaum
Library of Congress Catalog Card Number: 95-79047
ISBN 0-9647599-7-7

Published by Deva Press
139 Old Solomons Island Road
Annapolis, Maryland 21401
(800) FEEL-BTR
(800) 333-5287

This Book is Dedicated to:

My wife Rhonda, daughter Amy, son David, and mother Sabina
whose unconditional love made this book possible

AND

To my patients—
they have taught me more than I can ever hope to teach them!

Contents

Appendices

Patient Instruction Sheets

Resources

Acknowledgements

THERE ARE SO MANY SPECIAL PEOPLE who made this book possible that it is impossible to list them all. In truth, I've created nothing new—simply a synthesis of an incredible amount of work done by an army of hard working and courageous physicians and healers.

I would first and foremost like to thank my staff. It is their hard work, compassion, and dedication (and, I must admit, patience with me) that has made this work possible.

My research partner and lab manager, Birdie (Barbara Bird). Her sense of humor and encouragement kept me going when I got tired! Her dedication to quality shows in every facet of her work. Pat Miller was especially gracious, making sure that everything went as smoothly as possible. The hospital librarian, Joyce Richmond. Over the last 15 years, I've wondered when she would politely tell me to stop asking for so many studies. It's never happened—she always smiles when I ask her for more. My transcriptionist, Laurie Spangler, CMT, who patiently put up with my mumbling and repeated rewrites. Judith O'Callaghan, my editor and production coordinator, whose combined talent and dedication made this the best book it could be. Anne Masters Design, Inc., whose excellent design made this book so readable and beautiful.

9

My physician associates—Drs. Robert Greenfield (who taught me healthy skepticism) and Alan Weiss (who reminds me to reclaim my sense of humor!). My many teachers are the real heroes and heroines in their fields. Their names could fill this book. They include: William Crook, Max Boverman, Brugh Joy, Janet Travell, William Jeffries, David Simons, Jay Goldstein, Paul Levine, Jorge Flechas, I. Jon Williams, Leo Galland, The MAIP group, Leonard Jason, George Mitchell, Lloyd Lewis, Fletch Bartholomew, Art Schwartz, Michael Rosenbaum, Murray Susser, Paul Cheney, Alexander Chester, James Brodsky, Melvyn Werbach, Sherry Rogers, Byron Hyde, Robert Ivker, Jeff Bland, Alan Gaby, and Jonathan Wright.

The many CFIDS and Fibromyalgia support groups—these are easily the best patient support groups I've ever seen! I thank God and the universe for the guidance and infinite blessings I've received and for allowing me to be an instrument in its healing work.

Introduction
The Road to Wellness

Welcome!

I remember 1975. I was doing my pediatrics rotation in my third year of medical school. Having finished college in three years and being the second youngest in a class of over 200 medical students, I had always excelled. My approach to life was to move quickly—"full speed ahead." Then, a nasty viral illness hit me which made it hard to even get out of bed for my pediatrics lecture. Walking into an auditorium full of medical students, I remember the professor saying, "Teitelbaum, why are you…" As he said "late," I just about collapsed on the steps.

Although barely able to function, the next four weeks were spent working in the electron microscopy and research labs. These tasks were considered "low key" —a good place for a medical student to recuperate. By the end of the month, it was impossible to even get out of bed before noon. I wanted to push forward and try harder. Though it was not what I wanted to hear, one wise professor counseled me that this was not a time to push forward but a time to take a leave of absence and regroup. I am still thankful for his guidance.

My illness seemed to close a door to one chapter of my life and opened up whole new possibilities of self-exploration. Taking off in my '65 Dodge Dart, I had the novel experience of having no agenda, no plans. I was to meet many teachers on my journey. Most importantly, I took time to start to know myself.

With my family and friends' help and support and my own inner work, I recovered my energy and the strength to complete medical school and residency. Though doing well, I continued to intermittently have the many diverse symptoms seen in Fibromyalgia. My experience with Chronic Fatigue Syndrome (CFS) and Fibromyalgia left me with an appreciation of the impact of this illness. The symptoms that persisted (e.g. fatigue, achiness, poor sleep, bowel problems, etc.) acted as the arena in which I learned how to help people overcome the disease.

If you have Chronic Fatigue Syndrome, Fibromyalgia, or other disabling chronic fatigue states, you have been through a difficult journey. I remember being told that I was depressed. I was. I was unable to function. Most of us have had to struggle *just* to get compassion and understanding. Building on what I've learned since 1975, Barbara Bird (my lab manager) and I recently completed a study of 64 patients with disabling chronic fatigue. We have treated hundreds of others before and since the study. The majority have had complete resolution of their fatigue with treatment, while most others had significant, albeit incomplete, improvement. Only four percent had no significant change. On average we found it took patients less than seven weeks to start feeling better.[1]

This book will provide you with the tools and information needed to move beyond fatigue and into wellness. If you are a physician it will teach you how to, often dramatically, help your patients with chronic exhaustion—including the frustrating cases where no previous treatment has been successful.

Those of you who have researched CFS/CFIDS will find information here that is familiar and also much that is new. For instance, we have found that the key to eliminating chronic fatigue is to treat all of the underlying problems simultaneously. Most of you will have a mix of five or six underlying problems because of a vicious cycle where each problem can cause several others. You may have obtained some relief in the past from treating one, or a few, of your underlying problems. I think you will be happily surprised, however, at what happens when *all* of your underlying problems are treated simultaneously.

11

Certainly, there is much more to be learned in this area. Fortunately, though, we have now crossed a threshold to the point where we can effectively treat your problem. There are still many patients who obtain significant, but not complete, relief. As new information becomes available, we hope more and more people will join those of you who find that your CFS and Fibromyalgia resolves with the proper treatment.

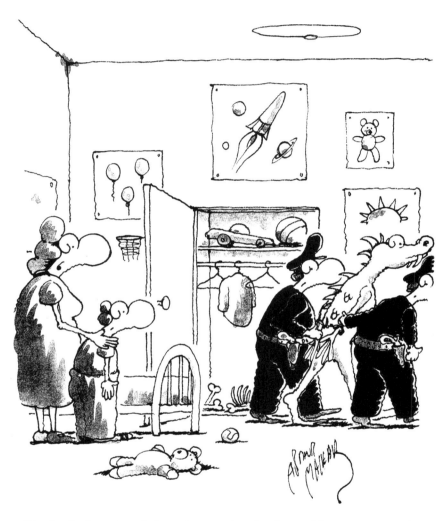

"And all that time I thought you just had a wild imagination."

1

Causes of Chronic Fatigue Syndrome and How to Get Rid of It

Chronic Fatigue Syndrome is a group of symptoms associated with severe chronic fatigue. The most predominant symptom or condition is that the person's fatigue has caused a persistent and substantial reduction in their activity level. There are also a number of minor criteria that are noted in Table 1-1. Poor sleep, achiness, "brain fog," increased thirst, bowel disorders, recurrent infections, and exhaustion after minimal exertion are some of the more common symptoms.

Table 1-1

UPDATED CDC CRITERIA FOR CHRONIC FATIGUE SYNDROME

A case of the Chronic Fatigue Syndrome is defined by the presence of the following:

1. Clinically evaluated, unexplained, persistent, or relapsing chronic fatigue that is of new or definite onset (has not been lifelong); is not the result of ongoing exertion; is not substantially alleviated by rest; and results in substantial reduction in previous levels of occupational, educational, social, or personal activities.

2. Concurrent occurrence of four or more of the following symptoms, all of which must have persisted or recurred during six or more consecutive months of illness and must not have predated the fatigue:

   A. Self-reported impairment in short-term memory or concentration severe enough to cause substantial reduction in previous levels of occupational, educational, social, or personal activities.

B. Sore throat.

C. Tender cervical or axillary lymph nodes.

D. Muscle pain.

E. Multijoint pain without joint swelling or redness.

F. Headaches of a new type, pattern, or severity.

G. Unrefreshing sleep.

H. Postexertional malaise lasting more than 24 hours.

14 December 94, Annals of Internal Medicine, Volume 121, Number 12 Table 14-1

The guidelines in Table 1-1 were put together by the Center for Disease Control (CDC). Although the CDC criteria helps researchers define groups for their studies, their previous criteria excluded all but about 5,000-20,000 people in this country who have severe chronic fatigue.[3,4] Unfortunately, over three to six million people in the United States alone currently have severe chronic fatigue states.[5] Research has shown that people with disabling fatigue who fit CFS criteria have the same immunologic changes and responses to treatment as those who don't.[6] My experience also suggests that the underlying causes and the response to treatment are not affected by whether patients strictly meet CDC guidelines.[7] I prefer to use the term Severe Chronic Fatigue States (SCFS) for these conditions. The symptoms and testing we describe below will help determine whether you have SCFS or other medical problems that require a different treatment.

14

We have found that patients who suffer from Severe Chronic Fatigue States usually have a combination of several different problems. The mix varies from individual to individual. There are, however, about 12 major underlying factors with each individual having an average of five to six factors. It is important to look for and treat all of the factors simultaneously. Chronic fatigue states are unusual in that each problem can trigger other problems. Because of this, it is rare to find only one single underlying problem by the time the patient seeks medical help.

The process that occurs is analogous to an automobile with no battery and no starter. If you fix only the battery or the starter, the car won't run. If both the battery and the starter are fixed at the same time, the car would be fine. In the same way, if we treat all of a patient's problems simultaneously, the person feels well.

Common Patterns

THE "DROP DEAD" FLU

There are several common subsets and patterns that we see in severe chronic fatigue states. The most notorious one is where a person feels fine and suddenly gets a severe flu-like illness that never goes away. This is a classic pattern for Chronic Fatigue Syndrome. In most of these patients, we suspect an underlying viral infection.[8,9,10,11] This causes an inflammation in the brain that suppresses the hypothalamus.[12,13] Hypothalamic dysfunction is also common in Chronic Fatigue States.[14,15,16,17,18]

What occurred when your hypothalamus gland was injured? When you had the severe flu-like symptoms, you felt wiped out, and you continued to feel both wiped out and achy. Because of the suppression of your hypothalamus, you developed an underactive thyroid and adrenal gland. The hypothalamus is the body's master gland; it controls most of your other glands including the adrenal and thyroid glands. A subtle but disabling decrease in the function of many glands then occurs. People can feel wiped out and have flu-like symptoms, however, just from adrenal gland suppression.

For most people, the suppression of the hypothalamus ended when the flu was over. Dr. William Jeffries, a Case-Western Reserve University endocrinologist, theorized that people who remained chronically ill after their infection had long term, or at times permanent, hypothalamic gland suppression. He found that by treating these people with adrenal hormone (in doses that are normal for the body), they often had marked improvement.[12] Our research has supported his findings.

What happens when your adrenal gland is no longer functioning properly? In severe cases, people can go into shock and die from even minor stress, such as having dental work. In most cases, the suppression is less severe, and the patient has moderate suppression of several glands. Dr. Jeffries showed how this occurs. In his excellent 1981 monograph, *Safe Uses of Cortisone*, we see that the flu causes suppression of the hormone (ACTH), which causes your adrenal gland to make adrenal hormone. Many fatigue symptoms are the result of adrenal suppression. When Dr. Jeffries gave fatigue and flu patients low doses of adrenal hormone, the flu-like symptoms often markedly improved.

15

Despite the glands being underactive, blood test results are often technically normal, albeit in the low range.[14] That is why many of you have gone to doctors and have been told that your thyroid or adrenals are healthy, when indeed they are not. Because of this, it is important to know how to interpret the tests and identify subclinical hormone deficiencies.

You may also have developed poor immunity, causing repeated bladder, respiratory, or sinus infections. I find that when people take repeated courses of antibiotics, they will often have overgrowth of yeast in the bowel. In addition, bowel parasites are also common in CFS.[7,10] The low thyroid and adrenal function and chronic infections can also trigger a problem called Fibromyalgia.

WHAT IS FIBROMYALGIA?

Fibromyalgia is basically a sleep disorder associated with shortened, achy muscles with multiple tender knots. Trying to sleep on the tender knots is like trying to sleep on marbles. Because of this, people have trouble staying in the deep stages of sleep that recharge their batteries. Instead, they stay in light sleep and often wake up frequently during the night. Finally they fall fast asleep; five minutes later the alarm clock rings, and they feel like killing it. In essence, if you have this problem, you may not have *effectively* slept for several years. When we restore normal sleep, people feel much better. I will note that sleeping pills (especially those in the Valium, Dalmane, and Halcion family) actually worsen deep sleep.

Fibromyalgia also causes fatigue by further suppressing the hypothalamus gland.[16] This results in immune suppression with secondary bowel infections. The bowel infections seen in chronic fatigue may also cause decreased absorption of nutrients and may increase your nutritional needs. This results in vitamin and mineral deficiencies. The hormone and nutritional deficiencies cause the Fibromyalgia to persist, and thus the fatigue cycle continues. Figure 1-1 "simplifies" this cycle (*See Chapter 14, "For Physicians," for an explanation of the cycle in more detail*).

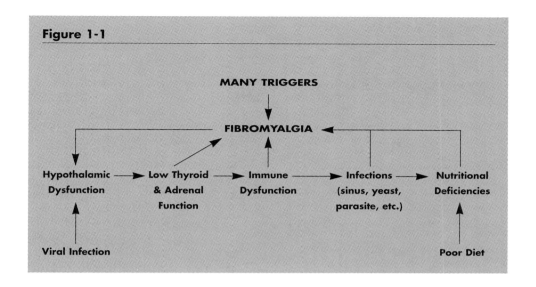

Figure 1-1

Many people enter the fatigue cycle directly through Fibromyalgia. Fibromyalgia may be triggered by trauma (such as accidents), by parasitic and other infections, and by chronic emotional and physical stresses. It can also be triggered by many other problems such as anatomic dysfunctions (e.g. one leg being shorter than the other) or jaw joint dysfunction (TMJ).

THE AUTOIMMUNE TRIAD

People can begin the fatigue cycle in other ways. These include autoimmune disorders where the body mistakes parts of itself for an outside invader. A common triad can occur where the body attacks the thyroid and adrenal glands as well as the cells in the body that help you to absorb vitamin B-12. The low thyroid, adrenal, or B-12 levels will trigger Fibromyalgia, which further suppresses the hypothalamus and the cycle again is set in motion.

You may find that you fit into one of the above patterns. There are many other patterns as well. When I ask the patient when the problem began, I will sometimes get the answer to the exact day (e.g. July 17, 1984). These patients usually fall into the first category of having an infection that suppressed their master gland (the hypothalamus). Other people will say, "Oh, the problem began about three to four years ago." These people most often have Fibromyalgia as a predominant factor with perhaps an underlying yeast or parasitic infection in the bowel, but this is also common in people who have the autoimmune triad noted above.

Sometimes we don't know where on the cycle people began, and, to be honest, it often doesn't really matter. I have now moved to treating the entire process at once so that people can get better quickly. There are trade-offs here, though. By treating several processes simultaneously, it is sometimes difficult to tell exactly which treatments are causing the main benefit. I feel that treating two to three processes at a time works best and, when the person is feeling well, we taper off treatments to see which ones are still needed. The choice of whether to treat two to three problems simultaneously or only one at a time, however, is a decision that is best made by you and your physician.

WHAT IT FEELS LIKE

Chronic Fatigue Syndrome and Fibromyalgia can occur in varying degrees of severity. Many people who have mild to moderate fatigue with achiness and poor sleep simply pass it off as aging or stress. Others have fatigue so disabling that they cannot even get out of bed, let alone do regular day-to-day activities.

The most common complaints that Chronic Fatigue and Fibromyalgia patients have are:

18

Overwhelming fatigue Most people with Chronic Fatigue Syndrome find that they are fatigued most or all of the time. Occasionally there will be periods where people feel better for short spans of time (e.g., hours to days). What usually happens then is that the person tries to overachieve to make up for lost time and, again, crashes and burns. Most often CFS patients will find that they wake up tired. This is especially true of patients who also have Fibromyalgia. The fatigue often also gets worse with exercise. When people try to exercise, they feel worse that afternoon and usually feel as if they were hit by a truck the next day. This, of course, causes further deconditioning and discouragement.

Frequent infections There is a large group of people who have recurrent sinus and respiratory infections, sore throats, swollen glands, bladder infections, and/or vaginal, bowel, and skin yeast infections. Some people get a recurrent red, bumpy rash that is resistant to treatment. They will often find this rash goes away for the first time in years when their bowel fungal overgrowth is treated. Abdominal gas, cramps, bloating, and occasionally alternating diarrhea and constipation are also very common. This has been attributed to a spastic colon and is often triggered by bowel yeast or parasitic infections. Poor food absorption and food sensitivities may also play a significant role in causing the bowel symptoms.

"Brain fog" This symptom is almost routinely seen. You may find that you have poor memory and occasional confusion. Your mind may seem foggy. This is sometimes one of the most frustrating parts of the disease and often the most scary. It is also a part of the disease that routinely goes away with treatment.

Achiness Chronic diffuse achiness in both muscles and joints is also very common. In most patients, this is part of their Fibromyalgia *(See Chapter 11)*.

Increased thirst When I meet a new patient with their water bottle in hand, I usually know what their main complaint will be. As part of the hormonal problems, people with chronic fatigue have increased urine output and, therefore, are a lot thirstier than most people. Drinking a lot of water is very important, and you may find that you need to drink two to three times as much as the average person. I would recommend using filtered water *(See Chapter 10)*.

Allergies Fatigue patients often have a history of being sensitive to many foods and medications. They can often get away with small doses of medications but may respond adversely to normal or large doses. Fortunately, severe environmental sensitivity is much less common. I find that food and other sensitivities usually improve when the adrenal insufficiency and yeast overgrowth are treated.

Anxiety and depression It is not uncommon for people with CFS to also have marked anxiety with palpitations, etc. The illness, combined with nutritional deficiencies, aggravates this tendency to anxiety and depression. These symptoms, as well, will often improve with treatment.

You may find that you recognize yourself and your problems in reading this. It is important that you know that you are part of a large group of people who have this problem and that you are not alone. There is an excellent national support group called the CFIDS (Chronic Fatigue and Immune Dysfunction Syndrome) Association. They are an effective support group helping to search for answers to your problem and are very worthy of your support. Their address, as well as that of the CFIDS buyers club and some excellent local support groups, is in Appendix I at the end of the book.

The good news is that new research continues to provide important clues on how to improve our treatment. For the vast majority of people with these symptoms, effective treatment is now available.

At this time, we will discuss the major causes of chronic fatigue and their treatment in greater depth.

Important Points

1. Chronic fatigue patients usually have a large number of other symptoms. Common ones are achiness, poor sleep, poor memory, "brain fog," increased thirst, and frequent infections. There are many others.
2. There is usually a *mixture* of underlying causes for the fatigue. This occurs because each problem triggers other problems. For example, hormonal problems (e.g. low thyroid and adrenal) triggers disordered immunity, which triggers bowel yeast, parasitic, and other infections, which triggers Fibromyalgia, which further worsens the hormonal problems. These problems are all treatable. People become well when the problems are all treated simultaneously. The mixture that causes *your* symptoms varies from individual to individual.

20

21

CAUSES OF CHRONIC FATIGUE

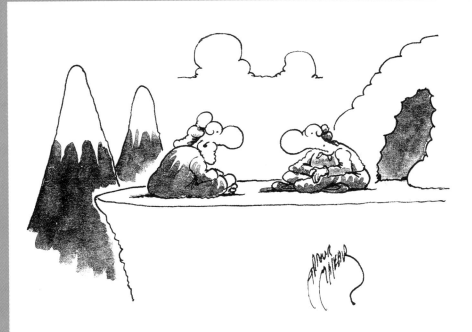

"It's the mystical balance of the universe. For every hotel towel you steal, a sock will disappear from your dryer."

2

Going After the
Easy Things First

Often people come in complaining of long-standing fatigue that is not quite as disabling as that which we see with Chronic Fatigue Syndrome and Fibromyalgia. I never cease to be amazed at how often people dramatically improve by simply cleaning up their diet a little: stopping caffeine, alcohol, excess sugar, and taking a good multivitamin. So let's start with the easy things first.

Poor Diet

The average American has over 140 pounds of sugar added to their diet each year.[1] This added sugar accounts for 18 percent of our caloric intake. If a good healthy diet without added sugar has only a 5-15 percent margin of safety for getting adequate vitamins and minerals, then the average American diet with 140 pounds per year of added sugar is already a disaster!

I often hear people say they are skeptical about the importance of nutritional supplements. They say, "Five hundred years ago there were no vitamin tablets, and people seemed to do just fine." Five hundred years ago, however, sugar was not readily available, or it was very expensive. The king of England might sprinkle a teaspoon of sugar on his food as a sign of power—but, if he wanted sugar, someone had to sail to the West Indies to get it.

Another problem is white flour. It is said that vitamins were first discovered by a Dutch settler who went on sailing expeditions with Dutch explorers. Soon after they set up colonies, he found that the people started to become ill. He also noticed that their chickens seemed to look unusually healthy. Being a curious fellow, he fed the chicken food to the people. Over a period of several weeks, people became stronger and healthier. He was a good businessman, so he (incorrectly) called the chicken feed Vital Amines (meaning vital proteins), which was later shortened to "vitamins."

We now understand what happened. It had become fashionable to polish off the rice's brown outer coat, or bran, and feed it to the chickens. Most of the vitamins and minerals, however, are in the bran. The settlers quickly became nutritionally deficient while the chickens flourished.

In the U.S. approximately 18 percent of our calories also comes from white flour—which has also been significantly depleted of vitamins and minerals.[1,2] Although some foods are now fortified with vitamins to make up for this, we are still missing *most* of the vitamins and minerals that have been removed.

As you can see, from just the use of excess sugar and white flour, we have lost up to 35 percent of our normal vitamin and mineral intake. Added to this would be losses from canning of vegetables (which can cause vitamin losses of up to 80 percent) and other food processing.[3] As Dr. S. B. Eaton notes in his study in the prestigious New England Journal of Medicine "physicians and nutritionists are increasingly convinced that the dietary habits adopted by western society over the past one hundred years make an important etiologic [causative] contribution to coronary heart diseases [angina], hypertension, diabetes, and some types of cancer."[4] This was the same conclusion reached by the authors of *Western Diseases: Their Emergence and Prevention*, published by the Harvard University Press.[5]

It soon becomes obvious that the argument "people didn't need vitamin tablets 500 years ago" does not apply to the average American diet. One study showed that less than five percent of Americans got their RDA (recommended daily amount) of all their vitamins and minerals.[6] What is frightening is that this study was done on USDA research center employees!

Each vitamin and mineral can be *very* important to your health. In addition, sugar may nurture the growth of yeast in the bowel and stimulate yeast overgrowth. Yeast grow by fermenting sugar, and they say thank you by making billions of little baby yeasties. Although most of the sugar should be absorbed before it gets to your bowels (where most of the yeast overgrowth is), most physicians working in this area have found that excessive sugar intake still markedly aggravates the symptoms of yeast overgrowth. Sugar can also aggravate the symptoms of hypoglycemia that are commonly found in people with an underactive adrenal.

Caffeine and Alcohol

I never cease to be amazed how many people who complain about being tired drink over ten cups of coffee a day. Caffeine is a "loan shark" for energy. Many people with chronic fatigue fall into the trap of taking ever-increasing amounts of coffee to boost their energy so that they can function. What they don't realize is that, as the day goes on, the caffeine takes away more energy than it gives. This starts people on a vicious cycle. It is a good idea to stop all of your caffeine initially for two to three months. You can then add back *up to* 10 ounces of coffee a day when you are feeling better. Caffeine is a drug. You may go through withdrawal.

If you are drinking more than three cups of coffee a day, start by cutting it in half each week (e.g. go from six cups down to three cups a day the first week, down to one and a half cups a day the following week, and then switch to tea with some caffeine). I usually tell my patients that I do not want to see them for ten days after they stop the coffee and sugar, because they are going to be grouchy and feel awful. Once they finish their withdrawal, however, they usually feel much, much better and are very happy that they did it. By tapering the coffee the way I described, it may take a little longer to feel well, but the withdrawal symptoms (e.g. headache and fatigue) won't be as severe.

Limit alcohol to one to two drinks a day (one drink equals six ounces of wine, 12 ounces of beer or one-and-a-half ounces of whiskey). If you are drinking more than this now, I would stop drinking alcohol totally for three months. If you decide to resume alcohol, two drinks a day is the limit. Many people with fatigue find that any alcohol is too much.

Vitamin and Mineral Supplements

The body is dependent on vitamins and minerals in the diet because it can't make them. Although I am going to talk more in depth about vitamins and minerals in the next chapter, I will simply note here that taking a good B-complex (approximately 25 mg) with minerals can have a dramatic effect on improving your sense of well-being. You will find your urine is bright yellow from the B-vitamins. This is normal.

I recommend that almost all of my chronic fatigue patients take an excellent multivitamin called TwinLab Daily One Caps with iron. This can be found in most health food stores or through the CFIDS Buyers Club. I recommend this brand since not all vitamins are created equal and many are poorly made. If you have a high risk of heart disease, such as a strong family history or high cholesterol, it is best to take the vitamin without iron unless your blood test shows your iron to be low.

I also recommend taking magnesium chloride, magnesium lactate, or magnesium malate, two tabs two to three times per day. This helps both the lack of energy and the achiness. If diarrhea and cramps are not a problem, you can take up to 12 tablets a day. Magnesium chloride or lactate is available from your pharmacy (over-the-counter without a prescription). Ask for Slow-Mag or Mag-Tab SR. If you ask your health food store for magnesium *chloride*, it will be one-half the cost of the Slow-Mag. The best form to take is magnesium malate, which is also available through the CFIDS buyers club, To Your Health, or Optimox (*See Appendix K*). If you get diarrhea from the magnesium, cut back on the dose. Take the magnesium for eight to ten months (it can take this long to replace your deficits). I would not take magnesium if you have kidney failure (i.e. a creatinine over 1.6, which is very rare in CFIDS patients. If the creatinine is 1.5 to 1.6, I would only take two a day for two to three months. Discuss this with your physician to get his or her approval).

The main side effect of the TwinLab Daily One Caps is an upset stomach in a small percentage of people. If this is a problem, try taking it with meals or at bedtime. If the discomfort persists, take a Centrum in the morning and a B-Complex vitamin 25-50 mg at a different time of day. If you still have problems (which is rare) experiment with different vitamins to see which ones your stomach will tolerate.

Exercise

Exercise is very important for your sense of well-being. People with Fibromyalgia often find that when they exercise, they feel wiped out the next day. Because of this they begin a vicious cycle where they are not able to exercise, and they become further deconditioned. The good news is that as you treat your problems you will go from being wiped out after exercise to feeling "good tired" for a couple of hours and feeling *better* the next day.

As you start to improve, slowly increase your exercise with a walking program. If you feel wiped out the next day, you pushed too hard, so ease back a little the next time. In time, you will find your exercise ability and stamina will normalize. Give yourself time, though, to *slowly* build up—you may have been deconditioned by many years of not exercising. The exercise, however, is important.

Many CFS patients have a sense of powerlessness and inability to defend themselves. Although the idea of doing martial arts (e.g. karate) training may seem impossible to you now, I think you'll be pleasantly surprised at your ability to do this training when your symptoms resolve.

I would exercise initially by walking, so you can get fresh air at the same time. Although getting fresh air may seem like a silly point, it is important. When the weather is chilly, walk in the malls or, as you improve, use a stationery exercise bike or a NordicTrack-type machine. There are cheaper ones that work fine. Swimming also can be very helpful.

Be Gentle With Yourself

People who develop severe chronic fatigue states are often Type A individuals who were overachievers before they got ill. As they start to get better, they have a tendency to try and make up for lost time and to try to get everything done that they couldn't for the last three to ten years. *DON'T*. Initially, use the energy that you get back to start doing things that feel good. Most of the things that have been built up over time can go *without* ever being done. *LET THEM*. As you start feeling better, take your time adding in new things. Pick and choose those things that you really want to be doing. Don't go "shoulding" (should do this, should do that) on yourself.

Important Points

1. Stop caffeine; avoid more than one to two drinks of alcohol daily.
2. Stop sugar.
3. When convenient, use whole grains instead of white flour. Add fresh fruits and vegetables.
4. Take a 25 mg B-Complex vitamin with minerals (e.g. TwinLab Daily One Caps vitamin) each morning.
5. Take magnesium chloride or lactate (approximately 60 mg tabs) or, preferably, magnesium with malic acid two tablets three times a day. Plain magnesium oxide (500 mg a day) is cheaper, but it may not be absorbed well.
6. When able, begin a walking program.
7. Get fresh air.
8. Don't try to make up for lost time as you start feeling better.

29

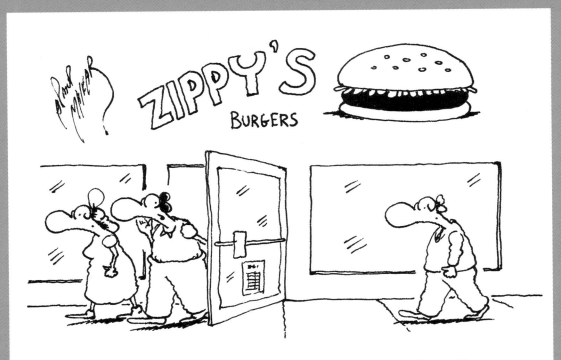

"Keep walking and don't look back, Phyllis. It's our doctor!"

3

Nutritional Problems

In Chapter 2, we gave an initial overview of the role of nutritional problems in Chronic Fatigue. A good multivitamin (e.g. TwinLab Daily One Caps vitamin) is critical to your improvement. If you have trouble with upset stomach because of the TwinLab vitamin, taking it with dinner or switching to a Centrum in the morning and a B-complex vitamin later in the day can be helpful.

Why are the vitamins so important? If you are low in vitamins and minerals, especially the B vitamins, iron, and magnesium, your Fibromyalgia simply will not subside. Dr. Janet Travell was the White House physician for presidents John F. Kennedy and Lyndon B. Johnson and is now a professor emeritus of internal medicine at George Washington University. In *The Trigger Point Manual*—her excellent book on muscle problems—she and her co-author, Dr. David Simons, have a wonderful chapter on perpetuating factors that cause muscle disorders to persist. This chapter alone has 317 reference studies on how problems such as hormonal, vitamin, and mineral deficiencies can contribute to muscle disorders.[1] We will discuss this at greater length in Chapter 11—Fibromyalgia.

Numerous studies show that adequate vitamins and minerals, especially folic acid and zinc, are critical for proper immune function (i.e. to defend against infections). Vitamin B-6, iron, vitamin E, vitamin A, beta carotene, vitamin C, and many other nutrients have also been found to be very important in keeping your body's defenses strong.[2-7]

Magnesium alone is involved in over 82 different body functions and is routinely low in the American diet (because of food processing). The average American diet supplies less than 300 mg per day of magnesium while the average Asian diet supplies over 600 mg a day.[8,9] If you take six magnesium lactate, or chloride, or magnesium malate tablets per day, you will only be bringing your dietary magnesium level up to normal. If your magnesium is low, your muscles will stay in spasm, and the Fibromyalgia will not resolve. That is one of the many things that makes magnesium so critical here. In addition, the magnesium is important for your muscle's and body's strength and energy.[8] Magnesium blood tests, however, will not drop below normal until *severe* magnesium depletion occurs.[10]

Iron is also important. Even if you are not anemic, an iron level that is too high or too low can cause fatigue,[1] poor immune function,[4,5,12] cold intolerance, decreased thyroid function, and poor memory.[13,14] I routinely recommend that people have iron, TIBC, and ferritin blood levels (three measures of iron status) checked if they are having chronic fatigue. Some of the insurance companies may balk at this, but the data and our clinical experience strongly supports doing the tests. If iron levels are even on the low side of normal, people will find that they often will be fatigued—even without anemia. Technically, your iron is normal if your ferritin (iron storage) level is over 18. If you have even minimal inflammation though, (e.g. a bladder infection) the ferritin measurement will be falsely elevated, and will falsely appear to be normal. Therefore, it helps to check all three tests for iron deficiency.

One report showed that females with infertility whose ferritin levels were between 20 and 40 (i.e. technically normal) often got pregnant when they took supplemental iron.[15] These studies suggest that levels considered normal to prevent anemia are often inadequate for other body functions. Because of this, it is worth considering treating anybody whose ferritin level is less than 40 (or whose "percent saturation" is less than 20 percent) with a trial of iron therapy.

We also find a surprisingly high number of people who have early hemochromatosis on their iron studies. Hemochromatosis is a disease of excess iron. In its early state, fatigue is often the only symptom. If caught early, it is remarkably easy to treat; if caught late, it is disabling and fatal. This is another reason to check the iron level carefully.

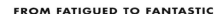

Vitamin B-12 is a key nutrient in CFS. Technically, the B-12 level is normal if it is over 208 pg/dl. Studies, however, show that people can get severe and sometimes long-term nerve and brain damage from B-12 deficiency with levels even as high as 300.[16] The question arises then as to why the normal levels are set so low. In part, this is because the levels were initially based on preventing anemia. We find that the brain's and nervous system's needs for vitamin B-12 are often much higher than that of the bone marrow. Also, much as I hate to admit it, the medical establishment has taken great fun and pride in holding in disdain the old-time doctors who gave B-12 shots for fatigue. The use of B-12 shots despite "normal" levels was used almost as a symbol for unscientific, old-time medicine.

As noted in an editorial in The New England Journal of Medicine,[17] we now find that the old-time doctors may have been right, and we were wrong. I suspect that we are a little slow to eat crow. In Japan, for example, I've been told (although I've been unable to confirm it) that a B-12 level under 400 is often considered abnormal and treated. A recent study using the respected Framingham Data Base showed metabolic signs of B-12 deficiency occur even with levels over 500 pg/ml.[18] I will also note that people with Alzheimer's disease have an average B-12 level of only 472 compared to those who have confusion from non-Alzheimer's disease, whose average B-12 levels run 887 (e.g. people with strokes, etc.).[19] This and other studies suggest that many people need B-12 levels that are significantly higher than what we consider "normal."

Our experience has been that when their other problems have also been treated, people often respond dramatically to B-12 injections. If the level is under 540, I will treat with 1 mg (1000 mcg) shots each week. These are very safe and fairly inexpensive. Usually, I expect to see improvement by the seventh or eighth shot if people are going to benefit. I will usually stop after eight to ten shots. If the person's symptoms return after a few weeks, I will have them continue the shots every two to five weeks for an extended period of time. Most people find, however, that staying on their multivitamin will maintain their B-12 level.

Why would low B-12 levels be such a common problem in people with chronic fatigue? There are several possibilities:

1. Vitamin B-12 is important for repair of nerve injury. Evidence suggests that there is an inflammatory process (called myalgic encephalomyelitis) that occurs

in the brains of many people during the development of Chronic Fatigue Syndrome. In repairing this injury, the body may over-utilize vitamin B-12, and, therefore, not have enough.

2. If an autoimmune process (*See Chapter 1*) impairs the thyroid or adrenal gland, it often will also decrease the body's ability to absorb vitamin B-12.

3. If people are on a vegetarian diet they may not get enough B-12.

4. If people have a bowel overgrowth of yeast or parasites, or other problems with absorption, they may not absorb their vitamin B-12 properly.

    Whatever the cause, we have found that treating the patient with B-12, even if their levels are technically normal, has often resulted in marked improvement.

Although we have talked mostly about nutritional supplements, I want to stress that eating a good healthy diet is also important. Eat a lot of whole grains, *fresh* fruits, and *fresh* vegetables. You don't have to be an ascetic or have a diet that is impossible to follow. It just needs to be reasonably healthy, and you need to avoid sugar. The closer you get to an unprocessed diet, though, the healthier you will be.

Important Points

1. Take a multivitamin, preferably TwinLab Daily One Caps, one a day. (Available through health food stores or the CFIDS Buyer's Club: telephone number, 800-366-6056.)

2. Take magnesium chloride or magnesium malate, two tablets three times a day.

3. B-12 shots for a series of 8-10 shots (and sometimes longer) are very helpful.

4. Be sure your iron level is checked and treated if low or low normal.

5. Eat a good healthy diet that avoids excess sweets and has a lot of fresh fruits, vegetables, and whole grains. The less processed your diet is, the better. Raw vegetables have enzymes that may help your energy.

NUTRITIONAL PROBLEMS

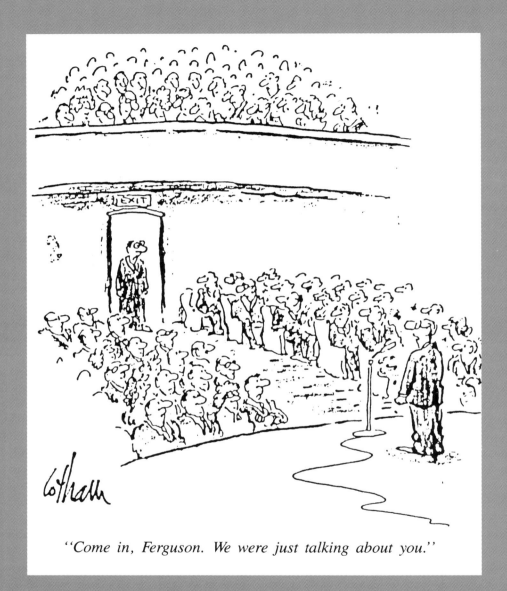

"*Come in, Ferguson. We were just talking about you.*"

4

Adrenal Insufficiency

About two-thirds of people with chronic fatigue problems appear to have an underactive adrenal gland. One cause may be the hypothalamic master gland not making enough of an adrenal stimulating hormone (CRH). I suspect many people also have adrenal "burnout." Dr. Hans Selye, one of the first doctors to research stress reactions, found that if you over-stress an animal, its adrenals will bleed and develop signs of adrenal destruction before the animal dies from the stress.

If you remember your biology from high-school days you may remember something called "the fight or flight reaction," which occurs during times of stress. In the Stone Age, when you met an animal that wanted to eat you, the adrenal glands would activate multiple systems in your body, and you would either fight or run. This reaction helped the cave man survive. In those days, however, you usually had a couple of weeks or months to recover before facing the next major stress.

In our current society, a stress reaction can be triggered every few minutes. Picture people driving to work and being late because of traffic; they are afraid that their boss will kill them. Every time they hit a red light or pull up behind somebody who slowed down, the adrenal gland's fight and flight reaction goes off. They get to the office; the boss is waiting for them, and it triggers again. They also have to deal with stresses at work including angry customers or difficult co-workers. Their spouse may phone, and they may have to deal with family stresses, and on and on. When people are ill, such as with chronic fatigue, another major stress is added. The different problems we discussed (e.g. infections, Fibromyalgia, etc.) put more stress on the adrenal gland.

I suspect that many people suffer a "burnout" of their adrenal glands—similar to the adrenal gland destruction Hans Selye saw in his experimental mice. With these kinds of stresses, the adrenal test may show hormonal levels that are actually higher than usual, as your adrenal gland overcompensates to deal with the stress. You may find, however, that your adrenal reserve (i.e. your adrenal's ability to increase hormone production in response to stress) may be diminished. Dr. Jeffries' experience, and ours as well, is that people with either low hormone production or low reserve often respond dramatically to treatment with a low dose of adrenal hormone.[2]

Dr. Jeffries opinion is that everybody with unexplained disabling chronic fatigue should receive a low dose trial of adrenal hormones.[3] Although he may well be right about this, I tend first to treat only those who "flunk" their adrenal test (called a cortrosyn stimulation test). There are different ways, however, to interpret the test, and I agree with those who are not as conservative as most in their interpretation.

What can you expect to experience if your adrenal gland is underactive? A low adrenal can cause:

1. Fatigue.
2. Recurrent infections.
3. Inability to shake off infections when you get them.
4. Inability to respond well to stress.
5. Achiness.
6. Hypoglycemia.
7. Low blood pressure and dizziness on first standing.
8. And other symptoms.

Hypoglycemia deserves special mention. Many people find that sometimes they get shaky and nervous, followed by dizziness, irritability, and fatigue. They often find that they feel better after eating sweets, which improves their energy and mood for a short period of time. Because of this, people will often crave sugar, not realizing that it shoots their blood sugar level back up to normal (initially making them feel better), but then their level continues upward. The body then responds by driving the sugar level back down, and this puts them on an energy "roller coaster."

Dr. Jeffries noted, and again our experience confirms his findings, that most people with hypoglycemia have an underactive adrenal gland. This makes sense when you realize that the adrenal gland has, as one of its responsibilities, maintaining blood sugar levels at an adequate level. The only fuel that the brain can use is sugar. When the sugar level drops, people feel very poorly.

We find that you can treat symptoms of low blood sugar by cutting the sugar out of your diet, having frequent, small meals, and increasing your complex carbohydrates such as whole grains and vegetables. Fruits (not fruit juices with concentrated sugar) can be eaten in moderation (one to two a day). Taking chromium (e.g. GTF chromium or chromium picolinate—250 mcg two times a day) for six months will often smooth out hypoglycemic symptoms.[4]

More directly, we found that the symptoms usually go away when you treat the underactive adrenal problem with low doses of adrenal hormone. I prefer using the prescription cortef instead of the adrenal glandulars that you find at the health food store. Their adrenal content is unknown and varies from batch to batch. One can easily become toxic from getting too much of the hormone.

But Aren't Adrenal Hormones Toxic?

Adrenal hormones are essential for life. Without them, we die. Like any other hormone, too much is dangerous. In the early studies using adrenal hormone, the researchers had no idea what dose was normal and what was toxic. When they gave arthritis patients injections of the hormone, their symptoms went away, and the patients felt better. If they gave many times more than the normal amount, their patients died of toxicity. The researchers then became frightened and avoided using adrenal hormones whenever possible. Because of this early bad experience, many of us were taught in medical school to avoid adrenal hormones entirely unless we had no choice.

To put the use of adrenal hormones in perspective, it is as if the early thyroid researchers had given their patients 50 times the usual dose of thyroid hormone.

Their patients would have routinely died of heart attacks. These researchers were fortunate enough to stumble on the body's healthy dose early on and did not have this experience. Otherwise, people would not be treated for an underactive thyroid until they became near-comatose (Myxedematous). We are just starting to learn in medicine that often people feel horrible and function poorly even with minimal to moderate hormone deficiencies. It does not serve them to wait until they go "off the deep end" of the test's normal scale.

Dr. Jeffries found that as long as you keep the adrenal hormone level within the body's normal range, the main toxicity may be a bit of upset stomach, (because the body is not used to having the hormone come in through the stomach).[5] If the adrenal level is low, people also may weigh less than the body's normal "set point" (even if they weigh more than they would like). When taking the hormone, their weight may go up a few pounds. This often is more than offset by the loss in weight that occurs when one is able to exercise. If an upset stomach occurs, the hormone should be taken with meals.

Your physician may not like the idea of your taking even low doses of cortef (adrenal hormone). In the footnote section you will see two references on the safety of low-dose cortisone.[2,5] Recently, studies have been published about bone loss with even low-dose adrenal hormones, but even these studies do not show significant bone loss at the lower doses that we are using.[6] Nonetheless, it is not unreasonable to take 1,000 mg a day of calcium with 400 units of vitamin D (e.g. Os-Cal 500 with D) or two cups of yogurt with live yogurt culture if one is on adrenal hormones.

If your symptoms started suddenly after a viral infection, if you suffer from symptoms of hypoglycemia, or if you have recurrent infections that take a long time to go away, you likely have an underactive adrenal gland. About two-thirds of our severe chronic fatigue patients have underactive or marginal adrenal gland function or decreased adrenal reserve.[1]

One other item of note is that licorice (real licorice—not the kind we find in the United States) and licorice extract can increase adrenal hormone levels. I don't recommend treating with licorice because everybody reacts differently, and it is difficult to be sure just how much of an adrenal hormone increase the person is getting. Although I prefer natural products to pharmaceuticals, I am more comfortable with the use of hormones (as opposed to medications). This is because the body can decide how much of the hormone it wants to use if the amount of hormone given stays in the body's normal range.

The adrenal gland makes many hormones in addition to cortisol. One of these is DHEA. We often find DHEA to be *very* low in people with chronic fatigue. Although we are just starting to learn about DHEA's function, it appears to be important for good health,[7,8,9] and it is worth treating a low DHEA as well. Studies show that the higher a person's DHEA level, the longer and healthier their lives. People often get a dramatic boost in energy on DHEA. If you have side effects (which are rare) start with 5 mg/day and slowly work up to what feels like an optimal level. I recommend keeping DHEA levels in the middle of the normal range for a 29-year-old (about 150-250 mcg/dl for females). The low end of the normal range is only normal for people over 80 years old! If facial hair growth or acne occurs (these are uncommon), decrease the dose. DHEA is available by prescription from Belmar Pharmacy *(See Appendix K)*.

Another important function of the adrenal gland is maintaining blood volume and pressure. Low blood pressure and dehydration are common in CFS. Recent research at John Hopkins Hospital in Baltimore suggest that a low dose of Florinef (.1 mg/d) can dramatically improve how fatigue patients feel. They suspect that the CFS patient's blood pressure precipitously drops at times (i.e. vasopressor syncope) and triggers symptoms that can last for weeks.[10] Florinef (a prescription hormone) prevents this. Begin with ¼ of a .1 mg tablet/day and increase by ¼ tablet every four to seven days up to one tablet a day. It can take three to six weeks to see the effect of the Florinef. Drinking plenty of water and getting enough salt is also helpful.

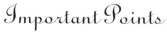

Important Points

1. Underactive adrenal function is very common in CFS.
2. If your fatigue began abruptly with a flu-like syndrome, or if you have hypoglycemic symptoms and/or you get frequent infections that take a long time to resolve, you probably have an underactive adrenal.
3. The best treatment for this would be low doses of cortef (adrenal hormone).

This is safe in low doses—and very toxic at high doses. Over time, the cortef dose can often be slowly decreased and eventually stopped.

4. Low adrenal function is tested by a cortrosyn stimulation test. There are many different ways to interpret the test. Often people are told that their adrenal glands are normal even when they may benefit from treatment. The varying interpretations of this test sometimes makes use of the adrenal hormone controversial.

5. Consider taking calcium 1,000 mg (with vitamin D 400 units) each day when taking the adrenal hormone.

6. DHEA (another adrenal hormone) and Florinef .1 mg/d (a salt and water retaining hormone) can dramatically benefit patients as well.

7. Drink plenty of water. If your lips or mouth are dry, you need more water. Be sure to get enough salt.

42

43

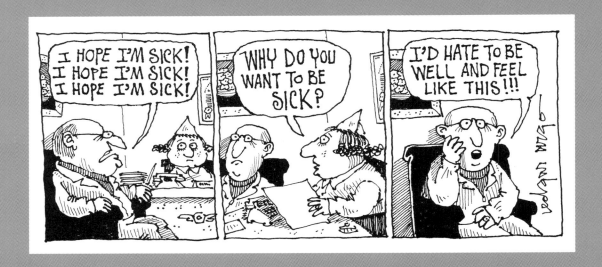

5

Hypothyroidism—
A Frequently Underdiagnosed Problem

The thyroid gland is our body's "gas pedal" and determines our metabolic speed. In medical school (long ago!) we learned to diagnose hypothyroidism by having people run on a treadmill while measuring their metabolic rate. We thought this was a wonderful new test and that we finally had found a way to discover exactly who had an underactive thyroid. We congratulated ourselves on being so clever and, then, the next test, measuring protein-bound iodide (PBI), came out. When we used that test we realized that, "Oh, we missed all these people with a low thyroid, but this new test will now pick up everybody who has a problem." We patted ourselves on the back and told all these new people who we discovered had a low thyroid that they were not crazy (as we had previously implied), they just had a low thyroid. We were comfortable and certain that we could now determine when someone had a low thyroid with certainty.

Then the "T4 level" thyroid test was developed. We realized, "Oh, that silly old PBI test. It missed all these people with low thyroid, but the new T4 test has now picked out everybody who is hypothyroid." Then T7 came out, and we realized we had missed the diagnosis in a lot of people who were considered normal by their T4. We felt certain that *now*, however, we had diagnosed them all. Then TSH came out, and we realized there were even more people with an underactive thyroid, but of course we thought we had finally diagnosed them all. We are now into our fourth generation of TSH tests and with each new test we realize we missed people who had an underactive thyroid. You would think we would finally catch on.

My impression and the impression of many other physicians is that our current testing still misses *many* people with underactive thyroid function. It is important to treat the patient and not the blood test. To make matters more difficult, if the thyroid is underactive because the hypothalamus is suppressed, the test can make it appear that thyroid function is normal, or even on the high side of normal.[1] That is why in the physician's section of the book (which I encourage you to read as well) I will discuss interpretation of these tests in more detail.

Suffice it to say that if you have symptoms of achy muscles and joints, easy weight gain, heavy periods, constipation, cold intolerance, dry skin, thin hair, changes in your ankle reflexes (called a delayed DTR), or your temperature tends to be on the low side of normal, and you have chronic fatigue, it is worth considering treatment with a low dose of thyroid hormone. As long as you don't have underlying angina (and most of you are not in a high-risk group for blocked heart arteries at this stage in your life), and you follow up with a blood test to make sure that your thyroid levels are in a safe range, an empiric trial of low-dose thyroid hormone is safe and often dramatically beneficial.

In some people, desiccated thyroid (Armour thyroid) helps when the synthetic thyroid (Synthroid) does not (and vice versa). In our experience, we found that about 47 percent of our chronic fatigue patients were felt to have a low thyroid either by blood testing or by symptoms and that 83 percent of these improved by taking a low dose of thyroid hormone.[2] If you have Fibromyalgia and you don't treat an underactive thyroid (even if your blood tests are normal), the Fibromyalgia simply will not resolve. This again has been the experience of many physicians who are very knowledgeable in this field.[3,4,5,6]

Some physicians recommend you check your body temperature for ten minutes each morning when you first wake up. Put a thermometer under your axilla (armpit) and lie quietly in bed. If your temperatures are routinely under 97.4°, consider a trial of thyroid hormone regardless of what the blood tests show.[4,6]

46

Important Points

1. An underactive thyroid gland is very common in chronic fatigue states. This may be the case even if your thyroid blood tests have been interpreted as normal.

2. Many physicians recommend a trial of low-dose thyroid hormone if your clinical picture suggests low thyroid (even with normal tests). This is controversial. Treatment with low dose thyroid hormone has been safe and frequently *very* helpful for my patients.

3. Symptoms of low thyroid (in addition to fatigue) can sometimes include cold intolerance, constipation, dry skin, achiness, and low body temperatures.

47

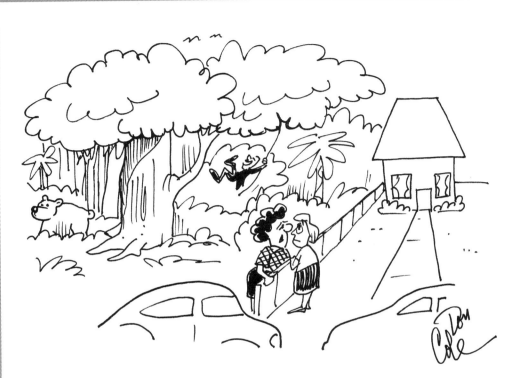

"My husband just doesn't believe in cutting the lawn anymore!"

6

Low Estrogen, Testosterone and Oxytocin— The Sex Deficiency Disease?

People often find that when they go through the change of life, be they male or female, they sometimes develop fatigue or depression. We find that if estrogen levels in females or testosterone levels in males are low, a trial replacement of these hormones can also cause dramatic improvement and is worth considering. We are also wondering if in females there may be a low testosterone level associated with an underactive adrenal gland, but we have never explored treatment for this. We will be beginning a study soon in which we will be comparing testosterone and other hormone levels in Chronic Fatigue patients (both male and female) with patients who feel well.

There is a lot of controversy about who benefits from taking estrogen when one goes through the change of life. Overall, the studies suggest that women who are prone to an increased risk of heart disease (based on high cholesterol, diabetes, family history, etc.), or osteoporosis, or have had a hysterectomy, will have longer and healthier lives if they take estrogen.[1] If one has not had a hysterectomy, progesterone (Provera) should be taken along with the estrogen to prevent uterine cancer. I avoid estrogen in patients who have been diagnosed with breast cancer. I am also slower to use estrogens if the patient's mother or sister had breast cancer.

If you don't like the idea of getting your periods again, the estrogen and a decreased dose of progesterone can be taken every day instead of cycling them. On this regimen, your periods will usually disappear in six to nine months.[2] Some people have found that using the natural estrogens and progesterones work better (and with less side effects) than the synthetics. This is an area I am just beginning to explore and therefore can not guide you on this at this time.

If the testosterone is low in males, I recommend a trial of testosterone shots, as men sometimes find that their energy will markedly improve. The shots are less likely to trigger cholesterol problems than the tablets. Testosterone patches will be available soon and will probably be better than the shots.

Drs. Jorge Flechas and Jay Goldstein, two physicians who do a lot of work with CFS patients, have found that many patients improve with oxytocin tablets (10 units/day-available through Belmar Pharmacy—*See Appendix K*). Dr. Flechas recommends that the DHEA level be brought up to mid-range (~150 mcg/dl) for three months first and that the patient take choline and inositol (available in health food stores) 1500 mg/d each for several weeks before beginning the oxytocin. There are no blood tests for oxytocin deficiency. Dr. Flechas feels that patients who are pale and have cold extremities are most likely to benefit from trying oxytocin. Although most doctors are only familiar with oxytocin's role in stimulating labor, it is also an important neurotransmitter (communication agent) in the brain.[3,4] If one is going to benefit from the oxytocin, it should occur in one to two weeks. I've been told that 10 units (the daily dose) is the amount the body releases each time we have an orgasm.[5]

Important Points

1. If you may be going through the change of life or have a decreased libido, check for estrogen deficiency in females and testosterone deficiency in males. If these levels are low, consider a trial of replacement with these hormones.
2. The effect of possible oxytocin deficiency is easily treated with oxytocin tablets (10 units/d). Consider a two-week trial (once your DHEA is normalized for three months) if you have pallor and cold extremities.
3. Your periods may be irregular for three to five months as you start to improve.

51

LOW ESTROGEN, TESTOSTERONE AND OXYTOCIN

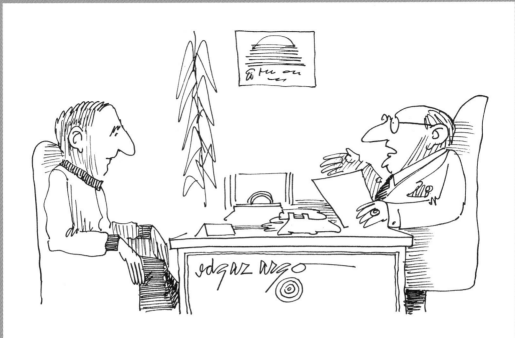

"*I'm of the opinion that we should operate…however, since you want a second opinion, we shouldn't operate.*"

7

Other Hormones

Clinical experience has shown us that some patients with diffuse hypothalamic and pituitary disease will not respond to treatment, even when their estrogen, thyroid, adrenal, and testosterone are replaced. Current research suggests that inadequate growth hormone may be an important factor in some fatigue patients.[1] A recent excellent study (currently being submitted for publication) by Dr. Peter Behan, a noted CFS researcher, shows that people with Chronic Fatigue Syndrome have a significantly diminished growth hormone level. Other studies have shown that low growth hormone can be associated with significant fatigue and CFS-like symptoms. These symptoms then improve with treatment.[2-5] In the future, growth hormone may help those few CFIDS patients who have not improved with our current treatment approach.

If you are lightheaded or drink more water than most people, it may be because your vasopressin (the hormone that conserves water) is also underactive.[6] Treat this by drinking a lot of water! In some patients, taking Florinef (a salt and water retaining hormone) .1 mg/day will sometimes dramatically improve all their symptoms and is worth a six to eight week trial.

Insulin resistance has also been reported in the later stages of CFS although I have not seen this problem. It was interesting to note that Dr. Jeffries found that diabetes often improved on treatment with low-dose cortisol.

The use of Florinef for fatigue states is still considered experimental. It is routinely used for other conditions and is felt to be fairly safe. Desmopressin (vasopressin) nasal spray is also occasionally helpful.

Prolactin levels are sometimes mildly elevated in our CFS patients. This probably has no effect on the patient and may simply reflect hypothalamic injury. Although we check an MRI of the head (to make sure no pituitary tumor exists) when the prolactin is elevated, this is usually normal.

As you can see from the preceding chapters, there are many problems that can occur when the body's master gland is not functioning properly. The good news is that most of these problems are easily treated. In our experience, treating these problems has often resulted in dramatic improvement. It is important, though, to treat the *whole* person.

Important Points

1. Other hormones may be underactive (e.g. oxytocin, vasopressin and growth hormone) or overactive (prolactin).
2. The effect of vasopressin deficiency (low blood pressure with secondary fatigue, etc.) can be treated with Florinef .1 mg/d. Consider a "therapeutic trial" for two months, if you have low blood pressure.
3. We've never needed to use growth hormone. This is fortunate—it costs $25,000/year.

54

55

OTHER HORMONES

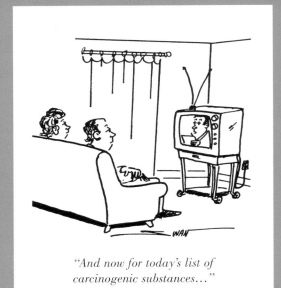

"And now for today's list of
carcinogenic substances..."

8

Immune Dysfunction and
Recurrent Infections

We have known for quite sometime that Chronic Fatigue Syndrome is associated with changes in the body's immune (defense) system. Although CFS is likely triggered by a viral infection, I suspect that in most cases the infection is no longer active. The body acts, however, as if the virus is still active. This results in elevated interferon levels.

Your body produces interferon to fight viral infections. When we give injections of interferon to treat problems such as cancer or chronic hepatitis, people develop achiness, fatigue, and a cloudy memory.[1,2] An underactive adrenal will also result in an elevated interferon level.[3] Because of this, it is more accurate to say that your body's immune system is not functioning properly as opposed to saying that it is underactive. Indeed, in many ways it may be on overdrive and will then exhaust itself. There are many other immune dysfunctions that are also seen, including decreases in the functions of "natural killer" cells, an important part of our body's defense mechanisms.[4,5]

When Your Defenses are Down.

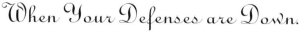

People frequently have recurrent and unusual infections because their immune system is malfunctioning. Chronic sinus, bladder, and other respiratory infections are common, resulting in numerous courses of antibiotics. This can result in a secondary yeast overgrowth, because the natural balance between bacteria and yeast in the bowel is changed by the antibiotics. Immune dysfunction also contributes to yeast overgrowth. Although this is controversial, many physicians feel that chronic overgrowth of yeast from the antibiotics is a potential and strong trigger for chronic fatigue, Fibromyalgia, and immune dysfunction. What makes this controversial is that there are no definitive tests to distinguish fungal overgrowth from normal fungal levels. Also, many of the symptoms ascribed to yeast overgrowth can come from the other problems we've discussed.

We frequently find that CFS patients also have bowel parasite infections. These can cause severe allergic and sensitivity reactions that can trigger the Fibromyalgia and cause fatigue. I will frequently see patient's long-standing and disabling fatigue go away within a week after treating a bowel parasite.

Many people have disabling fatigue following infectious Lyme disease and polio. Post Lyme disease fatigue and post polio syndrome also will usually respond to the treatments we have discussed.

How can one break out of the vicious cycle of recurrent infections resulting in repeated antibiotics, yeast overgrowth, decreased resistance, and more infections? This will be discussed in the next chapter on yeast overgrowth.

Important Points

1. An important component of CFS is disordered immune function. Your body may chronically think it is fighting an infection that is already gone, and this contributes to the symptoms.

2. Since the immune system is not working well, people get repeated infections such as sinusitis and other respiratory infections, bladder infections, bowel infections, and yeast overgrowth. These must all be treated while at the same time avoiding excessive antibiotic use.

3. Treating the hormonal, nutritional, and Fibromyalgia problems simultaneously often results in a dramatic decrease in infections, improved immune function, and an enhanced sense of well-being.

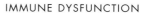

59

IMMUNE DYSFUNCTION

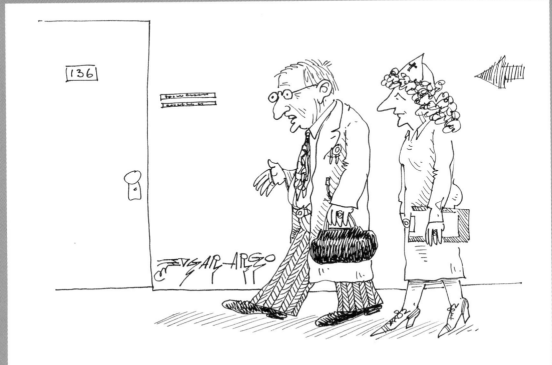

"*I'm just and old, country doctor…I don't hold much with all of this mumbo-jumbo about bacteria.*"

9

Yeast Overgrowth—
The Fungus Among Us

We all have areas of strength and weakness in our defense mechanisms. Some of us will never get a cold but may get frequent athlete's foot or other skin fungal infections. Other people may never get fungal infections, but have a tendency to bowel infections, and so on. Many of us have a diminished ability to fight off fungal infections.

Fungi are very complex organisms. Excessive overgrowth may suppress the body's immune system. The body may also develop allergic reactions to components of the yeast. Many physicians feel that a generalized suppression of the immune system occurs when yeast overgrow. In other words, once the yeast gets the upper hand, it sets up a vicious cycle that further suppresses the body's defenses.[1]

As noted in the previous chapter, this area is controversial. Yeast are normal components in our body's "zoo." They live in balance with bacteria, many of which are helpful and healthy. It is when this harmonious balance shifts and the yeast begin to overgrow that problems begin to occur. There are many things that may increase the tendency to yeast overgrowth. One of the most important causes is frequent antibiotic use. When we kill off the normal bacteria in the bowel, the yeast no longer has competition and will overgrow. The body can often rebalance itself after one or several courses of antibiotics. After repeated or long-term courses, however (especially if there is an underlying immune dysfunction), the yeast can begin to get the upper hand.

Many physicians have also found that sugar stimulates the overgrowth of yeast. Sugar is food for yeast, which they ferment in order to grow and multiply. The yeast overgrowth also seems to cause further immune suppression, which results in more bacterial infections and more antibiotic use. And thus the cycle continues.

There are several excellent books on the yeast controversy. One of the best ones is *The Yeast Connection and the Woman* by Dr. William Crook.[1] I find him to be a very concerned and caring physician. There are several very effective ways to take care of the yeast problem. First, avoid sugar and other sweets. It is all right to have one or two fruits a day, but avoid concentrated sugars including juices, corn syrup, jellies, and honey. Soda pop, which has 12 teaspoons of sugar per 12 ounces, is definitely out.

People will often go through withdrawal the first week that they go off sugar. This means they will initially feel worse and then much better. Many people have found that milk bacteria (e.g. acidophilus), a healthy bacteria for the bowel, helps to restore balance as well. Yogurt with live yogurt culture (e.g., Dannon or Stoneybrook Farms among others) is helpful. Indeed, a recent study has shown that one cup of yogurt a day can markedly diminish the frequency of recurrent vaginal yeast infections.[3] Nystatin, an antifungal medication, has been helpful.

Unfortunately, many Candida strains seem to be resistant to Nystatin, and the Nystatin in addition is poorly absorbed. This means that it will have little impact on yeast outside of the bowel. Other medications, such as Diflucan and Sporanox, seem to be very helpful here, although there are two main drawbacks. First, they are expensive ($450-$500 for a two-month course). Second, any effective antifungal, or anything that causes the yeast to die off rapidly, can initially make your symptoms worse.

If your symptoms are caused by an allergic or sensitivity reaction to the yeast body parts, suddenly killing off mass quantities of the yeast can flare the symptoms. This is especially true in people who have severe achiness from the yeast. Because of this, it is sometimes helpful to start with the acidophilus (4 billion units per day) and a sugar-free diet for a few weeks. I follow this with Nystatin (500,000 unit tablets or powder). I begin with one a day and increase by one tablet each two to three days until the patient is on two Nystatin tablets four times a day for three weeks. Then I add the Diflucan or Sporanox. I will usually prescribe one 100 mg capsule a day for one week followed by two each morning for five weeks. If symptoms recur after Sporanox is stopped, I would continue it for an additional three months at one a day. It is important that the Diflucan or Sporanox be taken with food, or you will lose much of the absorption. Do *not* use Seldane or Hismanal (antihistamines) with Diflucan or Sporanox. Also, if you are on certain antacid medications, such as Tagamet, Axid, Zantac, or Pepcid, you won't absorb the Diflucan or Sporanox. At $5 a capsule, I want my patients to absorb every last bit of it.

Once the yeast has been effectively decreased for six to 12 months, I feel it is acceptable to try adding *small* amounts of sugar back into the diet. If the symptoms recur, however, the sugar should again be stopped. Staying on yogurt with live acidophilus culture (unless you are milk intolerant) and/or the acidophilus capsules can also be helpful. I would note that your acidophilus should be the kind that was refrigerated when you bought it and stays refrigerated in your home. Otherwise, I suspect that all you are doing is eating dead milk bacteria.

Many books on yeast overgrowth talk about avoiding all yeast in the diet as well. This is based on the theory that an allergic reaction to yeast causes the problems. The predominant yeast that seems to be involved here is *Candida*—although I would not be surprised if we find that we are treating other kinds of fungal infections as well. The yeast that we find in most food (except beer and cheese) is not closely related to *Candida*.

In my experience, trying to avoid all yeast in foods simply results in a nutritionally inadequate diet and little benefit. Although there is a small subset of people who do appear to have true allergies to the yeast in their food, this only seems to be the case in about two to five percent of my patients with suspected yeast overgrowth (and these patients may benefit from the more strict diet in Dr. Crook's book). Interestingly, after I have treated the adrenal insufficiency and yeast overgrowth, most people's allergies and sensitivities to yeast and other food products seem to disappear.

Nutritional deficiencies such as low zinc and selenium may also decrease resistance to yeast overgrowth.[4-5] Your multivitamin should take care of these. As we can see, the factors involved are closely interrelated.

Important Points

1. Yeast overgrowth from repeated antibiotic use can suppress the immune system. This results in more infections, more antibiotic use, and more yeast overgrowth.

2. Yeast overgrowth may cause sensitivity reactions that are responsible for many of your symptoms.

3. To treat yeast overgrowth, avoid antibiotics when possible. Nystatin and other antifungals, especially Sporanox, can be helpful. Milk bacteria (yogurt and acidophilus) and certain natural antifungals such as caprylic acid often is useful.

4. Looking for microscopic evidence of bowel yeast overgrowth on stool tests is worthwhile. Unfortunately, though, there is no definitive test to determine if yeast overgrowth is part of your problem. Because of this, the decision to treat is usually based on your medical history and risk factors. (*See yeast questionnaire, Appendix C.*)

5. When you get respiratory infections, begin treatment with the directions in the respiratory infection information sheet that I give my patients (*See Appendix F*). This will prevent most respiratory infections from turning into bacterial infections that require antibiotics. For bladder infections, there is some evidence that Macrodantin causes less yeast overgrowth than other antibiotics.[6] Even with other antibiotics, most bladder infections will be knocked out with 1-3 days of antibiotics. Cranberry juice (*unsweetened* 10 ounces a day) or tablets also suppresses recurrent bladder infections.

65

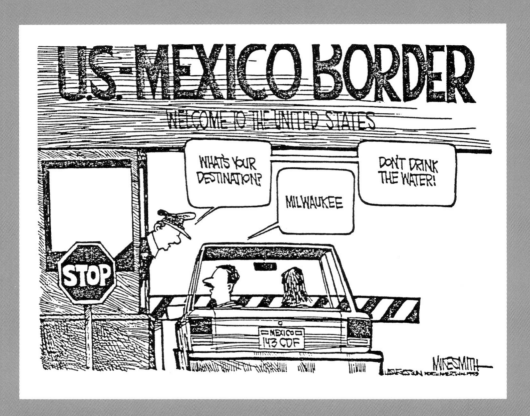

10

Bowel Parasite Infections

The news has recently focused our attention on Milwaukee because of repeated outbreaks of a bowel parasite called *cryptosporidium*. There is even a recent cartoon showing Mexican tourists being warned not to drink the water in Milwaukee! Although this bowel parasite usually goes away on its own within a week or two, this is not the case in people with immune suppression (e.g., AIDS). In fact, scores of people died from the *cryptosporidium* outbreaks.

Unfortunately, in many places the American water supply is contaminated. Parasites are no longer just a third world problem. We find frequent cases where people have infections with *giardia, amoeba, cryptosporidium*, and multiple other bowel parasites.[1] Parasitic infections can mimic CFS.[2-6]

Most labs will miss finding parasites on their stool testing. I initially tested for bowel parasites several years ago by sending stool samples to a respected local lab. They all came back negative, so I stopped testing for them. We now do the stool tests in our office. If done properly, this is a very time-consuming test, taking about five hours per specimen. We include both microscopic and chemical testing for different parasites. The result of doing careful testing is that we now frequently find people to be positive for parasites. Our experience and that of others is that when you treat the parasites, the patient's fatigue and achiness improve dramatically.[3-6] If you are going to have stool testing done, it is important that it be done in a lab that specializes in doing stool testing and that it be a purged stool specimen *(See Figure 10-1)*.

In a recent discussion, a gastroenterologist friend of mine noted that he saw thousands of parasites just swimming in the patient's large bowel during a recent bowel exam. He removed a big glob that had nothing but mucus and thousands of parasites and sent it off to the major laboratory in the city just to have confirmation and identification of the parasite. Even this sample came back as being negative for parasites. This is why we stress the importance of stool testing being done at a lab that specializes in parasitology. If you would like, your stool testing for yeast and parasites can be done in our lab *(See Appendix N for more information)*.

At this point, there is no good prescription medication for *cryptosporidium* infections. One of the benefits of having herbal treatments available is that there is an effective herbal treatment for this problem, *Artemisia annua*. We use 1000 mg three times a day for 20 days. Dr. Leo Galland, a parasite specialist, recommends a form of antemesia called tricyclin for many parasitic infections *(See Appendix K)*.

Filter Your Water

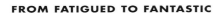

Water filters can be very helpful to fight parasitic infection. So I asked a friend of mine (Bren Jacobson) to research water filters. This is what he found:

68

To get a water filter that will remove parasites it is important to get a submicron solid carbon block filter. Consumer's Digest and Consumer's Report give the Multipure filter the highest ratings. For more information on this filter call Bren Jacobson at (410) 224-4877.

If you are considering another filter ask for the NSF International listing for the specific devices you are evaluating. NSF is an independent not-for-profit organization which tests and certifies drinking water treatment products. Filters should meet both the NSF Health Effects Standard 53 and the NSF Aesthetics Standard 42 (with class 1 reduction of chlorine and particulate matter). Any filter that doesn't meet both of these standards (particularly the health standard) is not worth the powder it would take to blow it up. To verify a salesperson's claims you can call NSF at (313) 769-8010. Ask for the Product Performance Data Sheet. Many states require that they be provided to all prospective customers of drinking water treatment devices.

Ask about the range of contaminants that the unit can reduce under Standard No. 53. Most units certified under Standard No. 53 are listed for turbidity and cyst reduction only. The number of units that also reduce pesticides, trihalomethanes, lead, and volatile organic chemicals is very small indeed. Be sure that the contaminants you are concerned about can be removed by the device you are considering.

Ask if the unit is licensed by such states as California, Colorado, and Wisconsin, which have some of the toughest certification procedures in the U.S.

Finally, ask about the service cycle (stated in gallons of water treated) of the devices. How often will you need to change the filter and what will replacement filters cost?

Important Points

1. Because of the immune dysfunction, bowel parasites are frequently seen in chronic fatigue patients.
2. People often *dramatically* improve when these parasites are treated.
3. There may be no bowel symptoms associated with the parasite.
4. Most labs will not find the parasite on stool testing, even if it is there and overt. Therefore, the test should be done in a lab that *specializes* in parasitology, and the sample should be a *purged* stool specimen. If you cannot find a local lab that specializes in parasitology, the test can be done by mail in our lab (*See Appendix N*).
5. Consider getting a good water filter that effectively filters out parasites (few filters do this).

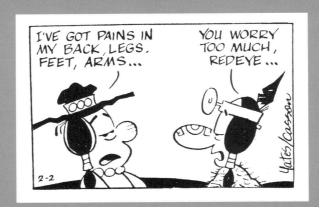

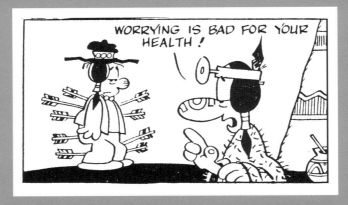

11

Fibromyalgia

ibromyalgia, often called fibrositis, is basically a sleep disorder with many tender knots (trigger points) in the muscles and other sensitive points. This is a major cause of the achiness that Fibromyalgia and CFS patients feel, and many people consider it to be the same as Chronic Fatigue Syndrome.

During sleep, we usually have periods where we stop moving and go into deep, very restful sleep. Unfortunately, in Fibromyalgia, the little knots in your muscles make it uncomfortable to lie in one position for an extended time, and it keeps bringing you back into light sleep. Because of this, Fibromyalgia patients are not staying in the deep stages of sleep that recharge their batteries. Although people with Fibromyalgia may sleep for 12 hours a day, they may have not effectively slept for many years.

Fibromyalgia is a cousin to other muscle diseases called myofascial pain syndromes. The diagnosis of Fibromyalgia is made by having 11 or more tender points in 18 specific locations (*See Figure 11-1*).

So How Do I Get Rid of It?

In their excellent 1300 page review of muscle pain, *The Trigger Point Manual*, doctors Janet Travell and Dave Simons review trigger points and their causes and patterns. They repeatedly note in their talks and books that it is important to treat the

Figure 11-1

AMERICAN COLLEGE OF RHEUMATOLOGY 1990 CRITERIA FOR THE CLASSIFICATION OF FIBROMYALGIA*

History of widespread pain

Definition: Pain is considered widespread when all of the following are present:

- Pain in the left side of the body
- Pain in the right side of the body
- Pain above the waist
- Pain below the waist
- Axial skeletal pain (cervical spine or anterior chest or thoracic spine or low back)

In this definition, should and buttock pain is considered pain for each involved side. "Low back" pain is considered lower segment pain.

Pain in 11 of 18 tender point sites on digital palpation†

Definition: Pain on digital palpation, must be present in at least 11 of the following 18 tender point sites.

- Occiput: Bilateral, at the suboccipital muscle insertions
- Low cervical: Bilateral, at the anterior aspects of the intertransverse spaces at C5-C7.
- Trapezius: Bilateral, at the midpoint of the upper border.
- Supraspinatus: Bilateral, at origins, above the scapular spine near the medial border.
- Second rib: Bilateral, at the second costochondral junctions, just lateral to the junctions on upper surfaces.
- Lateral epicondyle: Bilateral, 2 cm distal to the epicondyles
- Gluteal: Bilateral, in upper outer quadrants of buttocks in anterior fold of muscle.
- Greater trochanter: Bilateral, posterior to the trochanteric prominence
- Knees: Bilateral, at the medial fat pad proximal to the joint line

* For classification purposes, patients are said to have fibromyalgia if both criteria are satisfied. Widespread pain must have been present for at least 3 months. The presence of a second clinical disorder does not exclude the diagnosis of fibromyalgia.

† Digital palpation should be performed with an approximate force of 4 kg. For tender point to be considered positive, the subject must state that the palpation was "painful", a reply of "tender" is not to be considered painful. From Wolfe F et al: Arthritis Rheum 1990.[16]

72

underlying perpetuating factors that cause these tender muscle nodules to persist. Their 61-page discussion on perpetuating factors stresses treating nutritional deficiencies, infections, and hormonal problems. They also address in depth treating major structural problems such as one leg being shorter than the other or one half of the pelvis being shorter than the other (short hemipelvis).[1]

Appendix B is a very abridged version of their chapter. We have never ceased to be amazed at how quickly people's Fibromyalgia will resolve when these underlying problems are treated. The duration of the disease does not seem to impact on how amenable it is to treatment.

Fibromyalgia becomes self-perpetuating once it occurs. Even if the underlying trigger, such as a trauma that occurred years before, has resolved, the sleep deprivation may result in suppression of the hypothalamus.[2] Thyroid and adrenal suppression may be present despite the usual blood tests being normal.[3] The alteration of sleep can then cause fairly marked changes in immune system functioning.[4]

We have found that people will get well when you treat all of the major underlying perpetuating factors. It is important to understand that Fibromyalgia is both a common endpoint for many of the problems we have discussed and can also cause these same problems. The infections, nutritional deficiencies, and hormonal deficiencies can all, individually or in concert, trigger and cause a perpetuation of Fibromyalgia. Fibromyalgia can also cause the hormonal and immune dysfunctions and, perhaps by malabsorption, the nutritional deficiencies.

73

TREATMENTS FOR FIBROMYALGIA

There are many treatments that are both necessary and helpful for Fibromyalgia. One of the best known is to use non-addictive medications that increase deep sleep.[5,6] It often takes only tiny doses to see improvement, which is helpful as people with Fibromyalgia can be very sensitive to medications. I recommend either Elavil (amitriptyline 5-50 mg), Flexeril (cyclobenzaprine 5-20 mg), Desyrel (trazodone 25-150 mg), Soma (1 tab) or Ambien (5-10 mg) at bedtime. Often, it is like trying on shoes to see which one feels best.

I tend to use Elavil first unless the achiness is a very severe problem, in which case I usually begin with Soma or Flexeril. If anxiety is a significant part of your problem, I might begin with Desyrel first. Next-morning sedation (and sometimes

a lot—especially with Flexeril) often occurs when you first begin. This will usually wear off after two to three weeks. It is sometimes helpful to take the medication earlier in the evening (e.g., 7:00 p.m.) so that the next-day sedation wears off
earlier the next morning.

Health food store remedies, such as melatonin (3-6 mg) and/or valerian root
(180-360 mg) with lemon balm (*melissa officinalis* 90-180 mg), (*See Appendix K*) at
night improve deep sleep and are less sedating.[7] Ambien, (10 mg) at bedtime, also
causes less next-day sedation and in general has much fewer side effects. Overall,
I think the medications are more effective than the herbals for Fibromyalgia. If
medication side effects are problematic, using a lower dose (even ¼-½ tablet) *with*
the herbals and melatonin can help. For severe cases, especially if pain is marked,
Klonopin (.25 mg-1 mg) at night can have a dramatic benefit. Start with a low
dose and work up gradually because it is initially quite sedating. I use it last,
because it is mildly addictive.

It is critical that any nutritional deficiencies be treated or the Fibromyalgia will
persist. A high-level B-complex with minerals and magnesium are especially
important. See Chapter 3 for the supplements I recommend.

Gentle physical measures can also be very helpful. There is a form of neuromuscular education called Trager (developed by Milton Trager, M.D.) that has
been very helpful for our more severe Fibromyalgia patients. Most patients,
though, will not need these measures. If your Fibromyalgia were to persist despite
the treatments we have discussed in this book, I would consider calling the Trager
Institute in Mill Valley, California (*See Appendix K*). Ask if there is a practitioner in
your area, preferably a "tutor." The tutors have reached a *very* high level of exper-
tise in the technique. If you see a physical therapist, be sure you are seeing someone who is both good and gentle. We have seen too many patients who have been
made worse by physical therapists who were too rough with them. With
Fibromyalgia, gentleness is often much more powerful than being rough. If, however,
your body feels like it needs deep work, rolfing (*See Appendix K*) can be very effective.

Some people find that coenzyme Q-10 (a nutritional supplement that muscles use
as an energy source) can be helpful in doses of 30-200 mg a day. This is somewhat
expensive and can often be obtained at a discount through the CFIDS Buyer's Club.

Sublingual (under the tongue) nitroglycerin (.2 mg—ask your doctor to give you a tablet to try) can often dramatically ease the pain for three to four hours in about 25 percent of Fibrositis patients.[8] You may get a headache or lightheadedness the first few times you use it (so be sitting). The headache goes away with Tylenol and time, and often it does not recur. The first one to two doses should tell you if the nitroglycerin will work. Feel free to try the lowest dose that works (you can go up to .4 mg at a time). Have an eight-hour period each day where you don't use the nitroglycerin (e.g. while sleeping) so the medicine will stay effective.

Some people use aspirin-Motrin-like medications for the achiness as well. If this helps, it is worth using. Most people find using the Ambien, Flexeril, Soma, Elavil, or Desyrel to be effective without adding aspirin.

Treating the structural problems is also critical here. If one leg is even a quarter- to a half-inch shorter than the other, it can throw your entire gait off and throw your muscles into spasm. If one draws a straight line through the top of the right and left hip bone, that line should be parallel to the ground when both feet are together. If one hip is higher than the other, you will often notice that your shoulder on that side is lower than the other shoulder. This is your body's attempt at maintaining balance and puts a significant strain on your other muscles.

Finding somebody who does a good job with orthotics (a small shoe insert designed to make your hips the same height) can make a world of difference. I would consider seeing a chiropractor first (before getting orthotics) who does a lot of hands-on work (as opposed to one who only puts you on machines). You will often find that your leg-length difference goes away after a series of good chiropractic treatments.

If you find, when you sit, that the one hip is also lower than the other, putting a support under the low side so that the hips are even can often be helpful as well (the technical term for this device is a "butt-lift"). Often your chiropractor or a physiatrist (a physical therapy physician) will be able to help you in these areas. Rolfing (a form of body work—*See Appendix K*) can also be helpful for structural problems.

You will often find, when getting body work, that suppressed feelings and memories that have been stored in the muscles will be released. Experience, feel, and embrace these. Your awareness and experience (and then, if needed, releasing) of these feelings is an important part of the healing process.

Important Points

1. Fibromyalgia is a sleep disorder associated with multiple tender areas in the muscles. Medications that increase deep sleep, such as Flexeril, Elavil, Desyrel, and Ambien can improve the symptoms markedly. Herbal remedies, such as valerian root (180-360 mg) combined with lemon balm (80-200 mg), passiflora (160 mg), and/or melatonin (3-6 mg) at bedtime, can also be helpful if the medications are not tolerated. Klonopin, though moderately addictive, or Soma can be helpful in the initial treatment of very severe muscle pain (usually *not* needed).

2. It is critical to take a high-level B-complex vitamin with minerals (e.g., TwinLab Daily One Caps or the prescription vitamin Berocca Plus). Taking magnesium malate, magnesium lactate or magnesium chloride, six a day, (less if you experience diarrhea) is also important.

3. Treat the adrenal and thyroid deficiencies—even if the blood tests are normal.

4. Treat B-12 deficiency if your level is under 540 pg/ml. If you can't get the shots, take a 1000 mcg tablet daily (the shots work better). Take iron (not within six hours of a hormone, thyroid, or sleep medication) if your ferritin (iron storage) blood level is less than 40.

5. Treat the underlying structural factors (e.g. orthotics for short-leg syndrome).

6. Treat any infections—especially bowel yeast overgrowth and any bowel parasites.

7. Consider massage or body work (especially gentle, yet powerful, forms such as Trager and craniosacral therapy) if the problem persists. Acupuncture is sometimes helpful. Rolfing is also a helpful form of deep tissue work.

77

FIBROMYALGIA

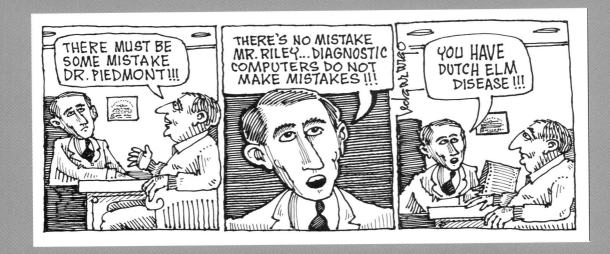

12

Am I Crazy?

n medicine, we have a bad habit. If the doctor doesn't know what's wrong with you, you're the turkey. Imagine calling an electrician if your lights didn't work. The electrician checks everything out, and says, "You're crazy, there's nothing wrong with your lights." You flip the switches, and they still don't work. The electrician just says, "I've looked, there's no problem here," and walks out the door. This is analogous to what many people with Chronic Fatigue Syndrome have experienced. I apologize for the medical profession's calling you "crazy" just because we don't know what's causing your problem. It is inappropriate and cruel.

What you have is a very real and physical illness. And, like most other physical processes (including diabetes, heart disease, cancer, ulcers, etc.), there is an associated psychological component. As with any disease, when we treat the physical component, it is also important to treat the underlying psychological issues. If not, the disease will simply manifest itself in another way.

It also helps to be aware that we sometimes mistake uncomfortable feelings (e.g. disappointment or sadness) for fatigue. Try to be aware of when this is happening. There is no such thing an inappropriate feeling. We have the right to feel whatever we feel.

Does this mean you are crazy? No. It simply means that, like all other human beings, we all have our emotional issues to deal with as part of our growth process. What I frequently see is that CFS patients are "caught on the horns of a dilemma" emotionally. They find themselves in a situation where they are unable to choose between two possibilities (for example, work and having children; staying with versus leaving their spouse; etc). These conflicts come in an infinite variety. Defending themselves against *acknowledging* the conflict then saps the person's energy.

Unfortunately, some patients have been so frustrated by being told their CFS is "all in their head" that they are in a "Catch-22." By acknowledging that they also have emotional issues (like everyone else), they feel they are validating the people who said their illness was all emotional. Give yourself permission to be human. You are no more (or less) crazy than everyone else.

I find that when people start to feel better physically, they find that it is easier to deal with their emotional issues. These issues are often holdovers from the past and are now easier to resolve. Actually, we don't always have to resolve our conflicts. If we have something that is irreconcilable at our current level of growth, it is helpful to simply hold the conflict in our awareness instead of suppressing it. Be aware that, "Yes, I have these two areas that are in conflict that I can't resolve now," and simply hold that awareness. The tension of holding those opposites while *staying aware* of the conflict will result in psychological growth (just like exercising helps a muscle to grow). You will usually find that, after a while, a solution will come to you from a new perspective.

A large percentage of my CFS patients are "Type A" overachievers driven by low self-esteem as a child.[1] In the first part of their life, overachieving was important for their growth and self-image. Although very difficult, the CFS has helped them slow down long enough to reclaim themselves. For many, a period of deep rest was essential. The illness has actually served many of my patients well. Part of getting well is "lightening up." The old Zen image of worry being "an old man carrying a load of feathers that he thinks are rocks" often fits. Many of the worries we carry will sort themselves out if we just let go of them. Although things may not always work out quite the way we would have chosen (CFS patients are often "control freaks"), they usually work out for the best. It helps to keep (or reclaim) your sense of humor!

I feel that psychological counseling is helpful to anybody who is growing. People who are emotionally and/or intellectually brain dead and living by the "social cookbook" instead of thinking for themselves may never need counseling. People who are in growth, though, will frequently come across areas that are difficult and with which it is usual and natural to need help.

Although many CFS patients feel depressed because of their illness, only a small minority have depression causing their fatigue.[2,3] "Depression" caused by CFS is often simply frustration. These patients usually have a lot of interests and are frustrated by their lack of energy. If the depression is causing the fatigue, the person usually has few interests. The stress of CFS can itself cause depression. Interestingly, the new antidepressants (Zoloft, Prozac, Paxil) often act as "energizers" even in the absence of depression. It is important to start with a low dose (e.g. Paxil 10 mg) and slowly raise it as needed. It takes six weeks to see the full effect. If the effect decreases over time, the medication Buspar will often restore its effectiveness.

Either way, it is important to find somebody who is effective to help you. Many psychologists and psychiatrists have never dealt with their own problems and are simply working out their own unconscious conflicts and issues on you. Others have worked through their own issues and are excellent. Talk to your friends and your physician to find somebody who is good. My own personal bias is to find somebody who takes a Transpersonal Psychology or Jungian approach. I have found one physician, Brugh Joy, M.D., to be extraordinarily skilled at helping people to understand their deep psyche.

81

Dr. Joy runs workshops up in the Arizona mountains. For people who are seriously interested in personal growth, I can't recommend these too strongly. They are a lot of work and somewhat expensive (although very reasonable for what is being given) and last approximately 12 days each. The workshop that I would recommend is his "Foundation" conference. I would not attend for the purpose of treating your chronic fatigue, however. I would go into it with the goal of accepting and understanding more fully who you really are. For registration and information, call Brugh Joy, Inc. (*See Appendix K*).

By using your Chronic Fatigue as a springboard for personal growth, having had CFS could turn out to be a blessing. I found this to be the case when I developed Chronic Fatigue Syndrome. It gave me a first-hand understanding of the problem and a powerful incentive to learn how to overcome it. It also has led me into wonderful areas of growth.

Important Points

1. Chronic Fatigue Syndrome and Fibromyalgia are definitely physical processes with physical causes.

2. All illnesses, including asthma, heart disease, ulcers, etc., have a psychological component.

3. Antidepressants such as Prozac, Zoloft, and Paxil increase energy in general. They are often helpful in CFS.

4. It is important to treat both the physical and psychological components of any illness. Getting counseling to help deal with the stress of CFS, as well as for personal growth, can be very helpful for anyone who has gone through the rough course that you have been through. I would recommend somebody with training in Jungian or Transpersonal Psychology. Twelve-day workshops with Brugh Joy, M.D. (*See Appendix K*), can be transformative.

5. Chronic Fatigue Syndrome teaches you how much you *don't* have to do.

82

83

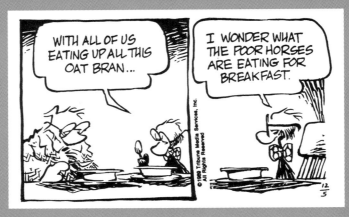

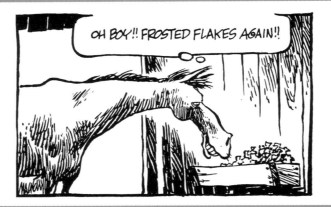

13

Other Areas to Explore

Although most patients get full resolution or at least substantial improvement in their symptoms with the approach we have discussed, there are some patients who still have a significant disability. There are important areas that are treated by other physicians but which I rarely get into. Many of these are worth exploring.

Food Allergies

I have found that most of my patient's food and other sensitivities resolve when I treat the underlying yeast overgrowth, parasitic infections, and their underactive adrenal gland. Occasionally, though, a self-help book on how to determine and treat your own food allergies[1] may be helpful. I use *How to Control Your Food Allergies* by Robert Forman, Ph.D. (recently out of print). Dr. Jeffrey Bland, a well-known nutritional biochemist, also has a very low-allergy food product for elimination diets that can be used to determine your food allergies. Although this costs a few hundred dollars, it is the most effective way that I found for people to determine food sensitivities and allergies. Information on the product can be obtained by calling Metagenics at (800) 648-5883.

Unfortunately, I have not found RAST or cytotoxic blood testing for food allergies to be very helpful. They are more expensive than the above approaches and incorrectly leave people feeling that they are allergic to everything. I have found these tests to be more crazy-making than helpful. We use a blood test that screens for ten common foods. It is more likely to be falsely negative than falsely positive. I would recommend an elimination diet as the best approach to finding what food allergies, if any, are present.

Another simpler approach is to eliminate the most common problem foods for two weeks. These are milk, wheat, eggs, citrus, sugar, alcohol, chocolate, and coffee. People with food allergies will usually go through withdrawal when they cut out foods that they are allergic to (i.e., they will feel worse for the first seven to ten days). Once they go through this "wall" they will often feel dramatically better if food allergies are a major problem. At that point, one of the eliminated food groups is reintroduced each few days to see which foods are causing problems. I leave those foods out of the diet and reintroduce them in a few months, as the sensitivity will often decrease. It is best to use these foods only every three to seven days initially and see how your body tolerates them.

There are many physicians practicing "Clinical Ecology" who use sublingual neutralization and other approaches. Although I am not familiar with these approaches myself, and they are controversial, I have seen many people get marked benefit from the Clinical Ecology approach.

Chemical Sensitivity

Clinical Ecologists can be especially helpful for people who have "multiple chemical sensitivity syndrome." I view this as a subset of Chronic Fatigue Syndrome, where the body has given up and is reactive to almost everything in the environment. Many people with Chronic Fatigue Syndrome have multiple allergies and sensitivities to environmental chemicals or different medications. Although this is common, it is *not* what I am describing here. Patients with chemical sensitivities are those who can't even live in a normal house because they become deathly ill if a new carpet is put in, if anybody sprays for pests, or if they come in contact with any of the thousands of chemicals we use normally. For those, I would recommend an excellent book by Sherry Rogers, M.D., called *Tired or Toxic* (Prestige Publishing, ISBN No. 0-9618821-2-3).[2-4]

Rare Infections—Mycoplasma

I have also found that there is a subset of people who seem to have infections with other agents that we have not been able to culture. After hearing from several microbiologists, there is one agent that is especially suspect in some people. Called a Mycoplasma, it is an infectious agent that is midway between a bacteria and a larger parasite. One that has been under suspicion as being involved here is called *Mycoplasma incognitus* (or *Mycoplasma fermentans*). There are some people who have found that when they take tetracycline for an infection, their chronic fatigue goes away for a short period. These patients, I feel, are at high risk of having an unrecognized infection, such as Mycoplasma (and should also be checked for sinusitis—see below). This agent is, unfortunately, resistant to erythromycin.

Doctors who are familiar with the problems caused by yeast overgrowth are very reluctant to use tetracycline, a major player in causing chronic fatigue states and yeast overgrowth (especially in people who have had many years of tetracycline for their acne). Despite this, if you have found that you have felt better after tetracycline in the past, or have recurrent lung congestion, or frequent fevers over 100°, I would consider a trial of doxycycline (a tetracycline), 100 mg two times a day for three weeks. If the symptoms improve markedly, this suggests that mycoplasma or sinusitis may be playing a role in your case. If the symptoms recur after definite improvement (especially if you have treated the other problems noted in this book), then I would recommend repeated courses of the doxycycline for two months at a time until the problem is finally eliminated. I would also take the precautions noted in the yeast overgrowth chapter while on the doxycycline.

Nasal Congestion and Sinusitis — A Commonly Overlooked Problem

Alexander C. Chester, III, M.D., a Washington, D.C., physician, has been a strong advocate of checking for nasal congestion and sinusitis as a cause of chronic fatigue. He found that many patients got marked benefit from following his regimen, even when they did not suspect nasal problems.[5] Fatigue from nasal problems is an area that used to be more recognized in medicine. Its importance is being rediscovered.

Dr. Chester recommends the treatment trial discussed in Appendix H. I would also add the regimen on the "respiratory infection information sheet" (*See Appendix F*). If improvement occurs on these regimens, consider using a cortisone nose spray (e.g. Vancenase) to maintain the effect. Sometimes nasal or sinus surgery may be needed. For those with chronic sinusitis, I strongly recommend the book *Sinus Survival* (*See Appendix L*).

Sleep Apnea and Restless Legs

Sleep apnea, where people stop breathing intermittently at night, often causes poor sleep and fatigue. It is most often (though not always) associated with being overweight and snoring.[6] It is diagnosed by having the patient spend the night being monitored in a sleep lab (although home testing is available). Restless leg syndrome (where the persons legs are jumpy during sleep) is also an important cause of poor sleep and will also be picked up during the sleep study.[2] These are both treatable. If you grind your teeth at night (bruxism), a mouth guard may help. The sleep lab should be able to guide you on treatment for these problems (*or See reference 6 and 7*).

People with loud snoring (or their spouses!) can be exhausted from the snoring (even without sleep apnea). A new surgical procedure can usually eliminate loud snoring (laser uvuloplasty). Your ear, nose, throat physician can either do this procedure or refer you to someone who can.

Seasonal Affective Disorder (Winter Blues)

If your fatigue is predominately from October to May, less on sunny days, and associated with increased sleep, increased weight and carbohydrate craving during the winter, you may suffer from sunlight deprivation (i.e. seasonal affective disorder—S.A.D.).[8,9] This is treatable with "sunlight boxes" (*See Appendix K for source*). Use a 10,000 lux box 18 inches from your face (at 45° angle to your face). Spend 30-45 minutes in front of the box each morning from September through

May. Add one-half hour at night if needed. Both sessions can be done while doing desk work, etc., and the timing and length adjusted to find the best response. If you have trouble waking, a bright bedside lamp (250 Lux) can be set (on a timer) to go on two hours before your wake up time. Portable light visors are also being tested. It takes one to six weeks to see the effect. Serotonin deficiency may cause S.A.D. Medications that raise serotonin (e.g. Prozac, fenfluramine) have been shown to be effective in treating S.A.D.[11,12]

Medications

Many medications have fatigue as a side effect. If you are on medications, especially if your fatigue has been worse since you started them, discuss alternatives (or stopping the medicine) with your physician.

Interestingly, a blood pressure-raising enzyme called ACE (angiotensin converting enzyme) has been found to be elevated in CFS.[10] People may have low blood pressure (e.g. from an underactive adrenal) despite this. Some physicians have noted that CFS symptoms improved in a few patients when they were given ACE inhibitors (e.g. Accupril) for their hypertension. Other studies show that some CFS patients improve with nimodipine or Calan.[13,14] If your blood pressure is high, a trial of nimodipine followed by Calan then Accupril could be a good choice for you. I would try each, one at a time for two weeks, and see which one feels best.

ALSO WORTH TRYING

Some people benefit from evening primrose oil, 500 mg 2 capsules four times a day (use Efamol or Linus Pauling Brands—many others are fake), plus Max-Epa (fish oil), 1,000 mg per day. It takes three months to be effective. The dose can then often be lowered.

High dose IV gamma globulin and ampligen (immune function enhancers) are being studied. These treatments cost *many* thousands of dollars per year, and I don't think most patients will need them. I do find that giving gamma globulin (gammar), 4 cc IM weekly (intramuscularly) for four weeks, will sometimes help patients with recurrent infections and is not expensive.

Kutapressin, a liver extract, can also help patients with severe recurrent infections. It's given 2 cc IM daily for three weeks. Then decrease the shots by one day a week every one to three weeks until the patient is on the shots three times a week. It takes three to four weeks to see the effect.

Magnesium sulphate 2 gram IM (by injection) weekly for four weeks is often helpful—especially if your achiness is severe and oral magnesium causes diarrhea. It is inexpensive but can be a pain in the bottom. (We add a small amount of novocaine to decrease this problem.) Some physicians give a lower dose of magnesium with B-12, B-complex, and calcium ("Myers cocktail") intravenously with significant benefit (especially if achiness, asthma, or migraines are problematic).

Coenzyme Q10, 25-50 mg three to four times a day, or a sublingual tablet 100 mg one to two times a day, sometimes helps (moderately expensive). This can be obtained through the CFIDS Buyers Club at (800) 366-6056.

Dr. Jay Goldstein, a well-known researcher working on brain chemistry and CFS, has many recommended treatments that can be helpful. *(See the end of Chapter 14 and Appendices M and L for recommended reading.)*

Our initial study *(See Appendix A)* for treating CFS/Fibromyalgia is scheduled for publication in the Journal of Musculoskeletal Pain in late 1995. We expect to begin our "double blind" study about the same time. Because of encouragement by the CFIDS Association support groups, research into CFIDS is increasing. Overall, the future for CFIDS and Fibromyalgia patients is very optimistic!

Important Points

1. Our understanding of the area is still evolving, and there are many other factors that may play a role in Chronic Fatigue Syndrome. Most people will get much better with the recommendations given in this book. There are many things worth trying that can be very helpful to those who don't experience full recovery with my initial recommendations.
2. Check for food allergies.
3. Treat for nasal congestion or sinusitis.
4. Consider testing and treatment for sleep apnea, restless leg syndrome, or snoring.
5. If symptoms occur mostly in October to May, consider light deprivation

(Seasonal Affective Disorder—S.A.D.) as a cause of your fatigue.

6. See a clinical ecologist if you have chemical sensitivities that are severe.

7. Consider seeing a well-trained acupuncturist and/or homeopath.

8. Are you on medication that may cause your fatigue? Consider trials of doxy-cycline if you have felt better in the past when treated with tetracyclines or have recurrent fevers and/or lung congestion.

9. If you are involved in litigation, the stress of this will often perpetuate Fibromyalgia. Moving beyond the legal case often makes it easier to get well.

10. Many medications can help improve symptoms of fatigue. These are reviewed in Chapter 14.

11. CFS is an area where research is increasing. Most patients can already get complete resolution of their fatigue, or at least marked improvement. Current research gives cause for optimism even for those who still have persisting problems.

91

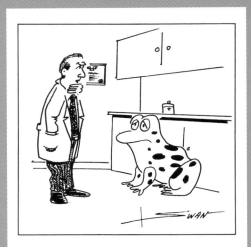

"You must realize there's a great deal modern medical science doesn't understand about curses."

14

For Physicians

The medical management of CFS and Fibromyalgia is, in many ways, fairly straightforward. Because the lab testing needs to be done and interpreted somewhat differently than you may be used to, I would recommend reading the rest of this book. If time does not allow this, reading my study on CFS treatment (to be published in the Journal of Musculoskeletal Pain—Winter 1995—*See Appendices A and B*) will help you to understand the rationale behind this approach, and give you a good overview of what is occurring in CFS. Four major physical components of CFS and Fibromyalgia are:

Hypothalamic dysfunction. This (or autoimmune injury) often causes adrenal and thyroid underactivity. Current evidence suggests that vasopressin suppression is also common. FSH and LH may also be low.[1-6]

Immune dysfunction. This has been documented in CFS.[1] In fact, CFS is now called CFIDS—Chronic Fatigue and *Immune Dysfunction* Syndrome. This may result in *recurrent infections*, often with normally nonpathogenic organisms such as Candida and bowel parasites.[7-8]

Nutritional inadequacies. Especially vitamin B-12, magnesium, iron, and B-complex vitamin deficiencies. These may be aggravated by malabsorption and increased utilization.[9-14]

Figure 14-1

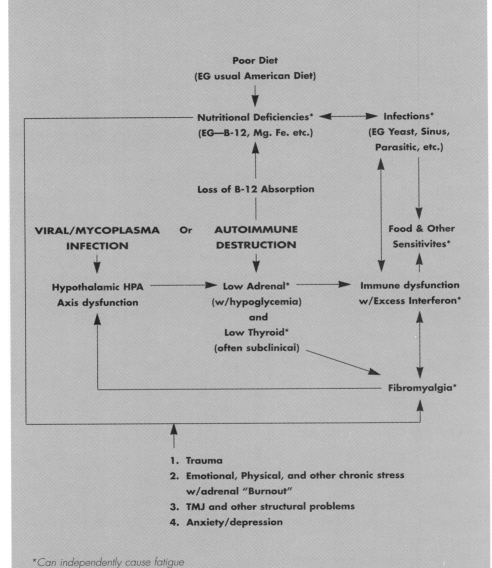

THE FATIGUE CYCLE

Poor Diet
(EG usual American Diet)

Nutritional Deficiencies*   Infections*
(EG—B-12, Mg. Fe. etc.)   (EG Yeast, Sinus,
                                Parasitic, etc.)

Loss of B-12 Absorption

VIRAL/MYCOPLASMA   Or   AUTOIMMUNE   Food & Other
INFECTION   DESTRUCTION   Sensitivites*

Hypothalamic HPA   Low Adrenal*   Immune dysfunction
Axis dysfunction   (w/hypoglycemia)   w/Excess Interferon*
                          and
                          Low Thyroid*
                          (often subclinical)

                                               Fibromyalgia*

1. Trauma
2. Emotional, Physical, and other chronic stress
   w/adrenal "Burnout"
3. TMJ and other structural problems
4. Anxiety/depression

*Can independently cause fatigue

94

Fibromyalgia. This is a sleep disorder associated with multiple tender points. Problems one, two, and three can cause and perpetuate myofascial pain syndromes and Fibromyalgia.[9] Fibromyalgia may also *cause* hypothalamic and immune dysfunction.[2]

These problems need to be treated simultaneously, as a vicious cycle occurs where each problem can trigger the others. Figure 14-1 shows the "fatigue cycle."

An Approach to the Chronic Fatigue Patient
SEE TABLES 14-1–14-4 (FOR SUMMARY)

I. HISTORY

Table 14-1 lists the symptoms and signs needed for the diagnosis of CFS. These criteria are more helpful as a research tool than as a clinical tool. In practice, the key questions are whether the patient has over six months of disabling fatigue, diffuse achiness that is worse with exercise, disordered sleep, "brain fog" (decreased memory and/or concentration), and perhaps increased thirst. If these are persistent and the workup has shown no other organic problems (e.g. anemia, cancer, diabetes, lupus, PMR or chronic infections such as sinusitis and Lymes disease), the approach in this chapter will likely help your patient. CFS and Fibromyalgia are not "all or nothing" problems. Like arthritis or many other illnesses, they occur in varying degrees of severity.

II. PHYSICAL

As with any disabling disease, a thorough physical is important. Look for palpable nodes in the neck and axillae. They should be smaller than 2 cm (if > 2 cm, some other process is likely occurring). Pharyngeal, nonexudative erythema is common. Clinically, several other areas of the exam are critical.

1. Figure 11-1 shows how to diagnose Fibromyalgia. It takes time and practice to become familiar with the tender point examination. Fortunately, the main clinical decisions determined by this part of the exam are whether to use one of four medications (Flexeril, Elavil, Desyrel, or Ambien) for sleep and whether an empiric trial of thyroid medication is warranted.

If the patient notes poor sleep and/or diffuse achiness, I would use one of the above medications for sleep, regardless of the exam. I would also consider a trial of thyroid (low dose) if these symptoms are present or the patient's basal temperatures are low. Have the patient check axillary temperatures for five to ten minutes each morning for five to seven days (before getting out of bed). Normal is over 97.4°.

2. Check for thyroid tenderness (thyroiditis is occasionally present) or even border-line thyromegaly. Check for a slow ankle deep tendon reflex relaxation phase.

3. Look for skin, nail, or vaginal signs of yeast or fungal infections. This would increase the index of suspicion for bowel yeast overgrowth.

4. Check for any nasal or sinus congestion, polyps, or septal deviation. If present, consider a trial of the sinusitis/nasal blockage treatment.[15] (See Table 14-5.) I also recommend the "cold information sheet" in Appendix F for respiratory infections.

5. Look for a "coated tongue" (as opposed to each taste bud being an individual white "dot"). This suggests B-vitamin deficiencies and will usually resolve after three to four months on a high B-complex multivitamin. Small 1-2 mm inflamed taste buds on the tongue that come and go are part of the same process. Tongue fissuring is suggestive of severe, longstanding B-vitamin deficiencies and takes four to five years to resolve (although the patient may still feel better quickly). A smooth tongue suggests B-vitamin and/or B-12 or iron deficiency.

6. Some researchers recommend looking for a "crimson crest" on the soft palate. This is so common in healthy patients that I do not find it useful.

7. Evidence of mitral valve prolapse is sometimes seen. Magnesium treatment is especially important in these patients (and is important even if MVP is not present).

III. LAB TESTING (INTERPRETATION AND TREATMENT RECOMMENDATIONS)

There are many approaches to lab testing in CFS. Some articles recommend doing very little testing, reassuring the patient that they're not going to die, and sending them home as untreatable. Not checking for treatable processes guarantees continued disability.

I recommend a fair bit of testing, but I limit it to tests that may help the patient recover. Many excellent physicians also check viral and immune titers (e.g. interferon and interleukin titers). At this time, these results would not affect my treatment or diagnosis. Therefore, I don't check them.

Table 14-2 lists the tests I find helpful. As noted in previous chapters, "normal" values may still need treatment. The interpretation of some tests is self-evident. How to interpret the others is critical to your patient's improvement *(See Table 14-3 for a summary)*. I have found the following tests to be useful:

1. Total T3, Free T4, and TSH. If the Total T3 or Free T4 are even on the low side of normal, I sometimes consider an empiric trial of synthroid, 25-50 mcg q.a.m., or Armour thyroid ½-1 grain q.a.m. I am more likely to try an empiric trial of thyroid hormone therapy if:

   A. the patient has Fibromyalgia.

   B. the patient's morning basal axillary temperatures are less than 97.4°

   C. the patient has symptoms and signs suggestive of hypothyroidism, and/*or*

   D. if the TSH is < .95 or > 4.0.

   We were trained to interpret a low normal TSH (e.g. .5-.95) as a confirmation of euthyroidism. The rules are different with CFS. In this setting, hypothalamic hypothyroidism is common, and the patient's TSH can be low, normal, or high.[16] This is why I recommend an empiric therapeutic trial of thyroid hormone treatment if the TSH and T4 are both low normal. Also, if subclinical hypothyroidism is missed, the patient's Fibromyalgia will simply not resolve. I would add four important points:

   A. If the patient does not respond to synthroid, switch to Armour thyroid and vice versa. (Synthroid 50 mcg can be switched to Armour thyroid ½ grain.) Each individual is different and can respond very differently. A low or low normal Total T3 would encourage me to try Armour thyroid (which has both T3 and T4) instead of synthroid (which has only T4).

   B. Adjust the thyroid dose according to how the patients feels and to get basal temperatures > 98° (as long as the T3 and T4 are not hyperthyroid).

   C. Do not give iron supplements within six hours of the morning thyroid dose, or the patient will not absorb the thyroid hormone.[17] Give any needed iron after 2p.m. and apart from any hormone treatments or sleep medications.

   D. Thyroid supplementation can increase cortisol metabolism and unmask mild adrenal insufficiency. If the patient feels worse on low dose thyroid replacement, they may have adrenal insufficiency.

2. Thyroid antibodies (antimicrosomal and antithyroglobular antibodies)—autoimmune and other forms of thyroiditis can sometimes trigger fatigue. Positive antibodies, and low normal T3 or T4 (especially with Fibromyalgia) strongly suggests that a therapeutic trial of thyroid hormone treatment may help.

3. Magnesium level—Serum mg++ will not drop until body muscles stores are at least 1/3 depleted.[18] (Perhaps equivalent to considering 2.8 to be the lower limit of normal on potassium testing.) I treat all fatigue patients with magnesium chloride or lactate (e.g. Slow-Mag or Mag Tab SR—available over-the-counter at pharmacies) 2 tabs p.o. t.i.d. Magnesium with malic acid may be more effective.[19] (Available through the CFIDS Association Buyer's Club, To Your Health or Optimox—*See Appendix K*). If the patient gets diarrhea, have him or her decrease the dose.

4. ESR—This is usually low (e.g. < 6) with Fibromyalgia and CFS. PMR mimics Fibromyalgia but will show a high sed rate, as will lupus, etc.

5. CBC with differential—If the MCV is > 93 in the absence of alcohol abuse, I would more strongly consider thyroid and/or B-12 treatment. If the eosinophil count is elevated, I would look more closely for asthma, allergies, and bowel parasites (although parasites are commonly seen even with a normal eosinophil count).

6. Fe, TIBC, Ferritin—We have diagnosed several cases of biopsy-proven hemochromatosis whose only symptom was fatigue (Elevated ferritin with a percent saturation > 50 percent would be an indication to explore this further.) If the ferritin is < 40 ng/ml or the percent saturation is < 20 percent, I would prescribe chromagen (a prescription iron), Ferrous Sequels, or Vitron C (if these cause GI upset) 1 q.d.-b.i.d. for four to six months (not within four to six hours of taking thyroid hormones). Although a ferritin > 9 ng/ml may prevent anemia, it may not be adequate for other body functions.[20]

7. B-12 level—Although technically normal if the level is > 208 pg/ml, studies show that severe neuropsychiatric changes from B-12 deficiency occur even at much higher levels.[21] Although current "normal" levels prevent anemia, they do not prevent neurologic injury. Recent Framingham data suggests that B-12 deficiency (determined by metabolic testing) can exist even with levels over 500 pg/ml.[22] If the patient's B-12 level is < 540 pg/ml, I recommend vitamin

B-12 injections, 1 mg (1000mcg) IM once a week for eight to ten injections. Although this is controversial, it is also safe, inexpensive, and often very helpful. It often takes about eight B-12 shots before patients see improvement. If improvement occurs but fades when the shots are stopped, I would resume the shots weekly until the patient feels better and then every one to five weeks as needed. It is reasonable to try an empiric trial of B-12 injections, regardless of the B-12 level.[23]

8. Stool for O&P, Giardia, C. difficile, cryptosporidium, amebic antibodies, WBC, and quantitative yeast testing. These are very helpful. We frequently find patients whose disabling fatigue *dramatically* resolves after their bowel parasites are treated. Although spastic colon-like symptoms are common in CFS, many patients with bowel parasites have no bowel symptoms. Because of the immune dysfunction, even treating parasites that are considered "nonpathogenic" can be helpful. Cryptosporidium (and other parasitic infections) can be treated with the herb artemesia annua 1 gm t.i.d. for 20 days. Dr. Leo Galland, a parasite specialist, recommends tricyclin 2 t.i.d. for six to eight weeks (Chinese herbal remedy, *See Appendix K*). Approximately one in eight fatigue patients test positive for stool parasites.

Although there is no good test for stool fungal overgrowth (making this a controversial area), we find that quantifying stool yeast levels (on O&P) is very helpful. *Most labs will not find parasites in the stool even if they are present!*[24] The patient needs to take 1½ ounces of a Fleets Phospho Soda laxative before the test and get three loose stool samples. Find a lab that *specializes* in parasitology for your O&Ps. If no such lab is available, the stool tests can be done by mail in our lab *(See Appendix N)*. We can then give treatment recommendations based on the results.

9. Serum or stool ameba antibodies—Cysts are passed intermittently and O&Ps may miss amebic infections. This is a helpful backup test. If amebic infection is suspected based on testing, consider Flagyl 750 mg p.o. t.i.d. (less if not tolerated) for ten days, followed by 650 mg of Yodoxin t.i.d. for 20 more days.

10. CPK—Screens for dermatomyositis, polymyositis, etc.

11. Cortrosyn stimulation test—Checks adrenal function. This is a critical test *(See Appendix E for patient instructions for the cortrosyn test and cortef treatment)*. This

test can be done at your office or by sending the patient to the lab. It is important that the cortisol baseline is drawn between 8 and 9 a.m. After checking the baseline cortisol, give 25 units of ACTH (cortrosyn) IM and check cortisol levels at one-half and one hour. I consider the test to be positive if:

A. The cortisol level at baseline is less than 6 mcg/dl *or*

B. The cortisol level does not increase by at least 7 mcg/dl at ½ hour and 11 mcg/dl at 1 hour *or*

C. The cortisol level does not double from the baseline and is under 35-40 mcg/dl. There is not a consensus on the test's interpretation. Many consider the test positive if any of the above criteria are met. Others consider any test where the cortisol level goes over 20 mcg/dl to be normal.

Dr. William Jeffries, a retired professor of endocrinology at Case-Western Reserve Medical School, has researched cortisol treatment for many decades in chronic fatigue states. He recommends considering an empiric trial of cortef, approximately 5 mg-7.5 mg t.i.d. to q.i.d., in all cases of severe, unexpected fatigue[25,26] for the following reasons:

A. Strict interpretation of the test misses many cases of disabling, suboptimal adrenal function.

B. The doses of cortef being used here are fairly safe.[27]

C. Patients often experience dramatic improvement with low-dose cortef in CFS.[26]

D. Hypothalamic-pituitary-adrenal axis dysfunction has been demonstrated in chronic fatigue patients.[1-6]

I begin with the following approximate guidelines:

If the baseline cortisol is	I treat with cortef
A. < 12 mcg/dl	5 mg t.i.d. with meals
B. > 12 mcg/dl but does not increase by 7 mcg/dl at one-half hour *and* 11 mcg/dl at one hour or does not double by one hour (and is < 40 mcg/dl)	5 mg in the a.m. and 2.5 mg at lunch and increase to 5 mg p.o. t.i.d. p.r.n.

After two to four weeks on the initial dose, adjust the dose up to a maximum of 30 mg/d or taper it off if there is no benefit. Give most of the cortef in the morning and at lunch. I often give the last dose (of 2.5-5 mg cortef) no later than 4 p.m. Otherwise, it can keep the patient up at night.

After eight to 12 months on cortef, it is reasonable to taper off the cortef over one to two months and repeat the cortosyn test. By eliminating the other physiologic stresses (infections, Fibromyalgia, etc), many patient's adrenal function will be adequate and/or normalize. Some patients require long-term treatment.

Improvement is often dramatic and usually seen within two weeks. The dose should be doubled during periods of acute stress (higher for severe stress—e.g. surgery). Consider giving calcium 1000 mg and Vitamin D 400 I.U. daily with the cortef.

Being a center for CFS research, an NIH research team has invited us to contribute patients for a currently ongoing controlled study using cortef in all patients with CFS (37.5 mg/d). Their group has done excellent work in CFS. My concern is that, by not treating the other factors causing CFS, they may miss much of cortef's treatment benefits.

12. Glycosylated hemoglobin (HgbA1C)—Although not very specific, I find it helpful to screen for hypoglycemia. Hypoglycemia is most often caused by inadequate adrenal function.[26] If < 5.2 it suggests that a trial of low-dose cortef may help even if the cortosyn test is borderline. The test also will, of course, screen for diabetes.

13. DHEA—This is a major adrenal hormone. Low levels are associated with shorter life (See Table 14-6).[28] If the DHEA level is under 150 mcg/dl (See Table 14-6 for normal ranges, which are based on patient's sex and age) I recommend a therapeutic trial of DHEA treatment. People often have improved energy when treated with DHEA 5-60 mg q.d.[29] (Adjusted to keep the DHEA level at least 150 mcg/dl.) DHEA levels should be checked six to eight weeks after dosing changes. The DHEA can be ordered through Professional Arts Pharmacy (800) 832-9285 or Belmar Pharmacy (800) 525-9473.

14. Chem 19 and U/A with micro—to screen for liver, kidney, and other metabolic problems.

15. ANA (antinuclear antibody) and latex fixation—to screen for lupus, rheumatoid arthritis, and other connective tissue diseases. These can cause a secondary Fibromyalgia.

16. Lymes, H.I.V., RPR—These infections can cause chronic fatigue and Fibromyalgia. False positive Lyme titers are common and must be confirmed by other testing and clinical setting.

17. FSH and LH—Check if menopause is a consideration. Early menopause, even with regular periods, is sometimes seen. Night sweats can interfere with sleep and cause fatigue. Treatment with Premarin has at times resulted in dramatic improvement.

18. IgE and allergy testing—If allergies are suspected.

19. PPD—To screen for TB.

20. Sinus CT scan—Consider if chronic sinusitis is present and persists despite Rx.

21. Sleep testing—If sleep apnea or restless leg syndrome are suspected. Sleep apnea is more likely if the patient is male, overweight, and/or snores.

22. In the future, testing for insulin-stimulated growth hormone levels may help in nonresponders.

23. Yeast questionnaire (See Appendix C)—There is no definitive test to differentiate normal yeast growth from overgrowth. Yeast overgrowth is suspected if the patient has a high score on the questionnaire or shows yeast overgrowth on the stool microscopic exam. An empiric trial of Nystatin 500,000 IU 2 tabs q.i.d. (start slowly) for five months with Diflucan or Sporanox 100 mg, one a day, for one week followed by 200 mg each morning for five weeks, is often dramatically helpful. The patient's symptoms (especially the Fibromyalgia pain) may flare initially as the yeast die off. Therefore, begin with Nystatin 500,000 units one a day and increase by one tablet every one to three days (as tolerated) up to two tablets four times a day. Some physicians feel the Nystatin powder is more effective than the tablets. After four to six weeks on Nystatin, add the Diflucan or Sporanox as above. The other major side effect of the Diflucan and Sporanox is that they cost more than $500 for 90 capsules. If symptoms recur after the first two months on Diflucan or Sporanox, I repeat one capsule per day for three more months. If there was no benefit with the first course, I don't repeat it.

Sporanox and Diflucan must be taken with food to be properly absorbed. H2 blockers (e.g. Zantac) will prevent absorption. Do not use Seldane or Hismanal with Sporinox or Diflucan (can cause fatal arrhythmias). Sweets must also be avoided—they seem to stimulate yeast growth. One cup of yogurt (with live culture) daily is helpful. Refrigerated acidophilus bacteria (4 billion units/day) also can help to restore the normal bowel flora.

IV. TREATMENT (GENERAL—IN ADDITION TO THE ABOVE RECOMMENDATIONS)

1. TwinLab Daily One caps (OTC) or Berocca Plus vitamin (prescription—Use generic since it $15 versus $50 per 100), one a day. This multivitamin turns the urine bright yellow. Have patients take it with food if it causes nausea.

2. Magnesium chloride (Slow-Mag), magnesium lactate (Mag Tabs SR), or, preferably, magnesium malate (from CFIDS Buyer's Club, *See Appendix K*), two tablets three times a day.

3. No sweets for six months (including no non-diet sodas).

4. No caffeine or alcohol for six months.

5. Work to uncover any life conflicts. I find the Jungian approach to counseling very helpful.

6. As the patient improves, have them slowly begin to exercise. Begin with walking and advance as able. If the patient feels "wiped out" the next day, they pushed too hard and need to ease back.

7. Avoid antibiotics when possible. Erythromycin and Macrodantin seem to cause less yeast overgrowth.

8. Sleep eight hours per night.

9. Encourage patients not to try to make up for lost time when they start to feel well. They may not be able to return to work even if they feel well.

For Other Problems (SEE SECTION II ON TESTING AND TABLE 14-3)

Fibromyalgia Treating the rest of the problems we've discussed is critical and often results in dramatic improvement in the patient's Fibromyalgia. Non-addictive medication to restore deep sleep is very helpful. Fibromyalgia patients tend to be sensitive to medications. It helps to start with a very low dose. The next-day sedation often resolves in two to three weeks. The medication can be taken earlier in the evening (e.g. 7 p.m.) so it wears off earlier the next day. I do not recommend addictive sleeping pills! These actually decrease the time spent in deep sleep and can worsen Fibromyalgia (except for Klonopin). I recommend using the following medications—adjust the dose so that the patient sleeps deeply through the night.

1. Elavil (amitriptyline) 10 mg—use ½-5 tablets at bed time.
2. Ambien—use 5-10 mg at bedtime. This is a newer agent that has less side effects than the other medications. It is very helpful in many patients.
3. Flexeril (cyclobenzaprine), 10 mg and/or Soma—Use ½-1 tablet at bedtime. Often very sedating. Use these first if myalgias are a major problem.
4. Desyrel (trazodone) 50 mg—Use ½-6 tablets at bedtime. (Use this first if anxiety is a major problem.)
5. Health Food Store Products—If medication is not tolerated, use valerian root 360 mg, plus passiflora 160 mg, plus lemon balm 160 mg at bedtime. Melatonin 3-6 mg q.h.s. is also helpful. Often adding these to allow a lower dose of medication can be helpful.

For patients with disabling muscle aches, Klonopin can be very helpful. It is potentially mildly addictive, so I reserve it for patients with severe pain who don't respond to or tolerate the other medications. Begin with .25 mg at bedtime and slowly adjust the dose upward.

About 15-25 percent of Fibromyalgia patients will get about four hours relief from their achiness with sublingual nitroglycerin .2-.3 mg (begin with one-half tablet or less). The initial headache usually goes away after the first few tablets. Massage and *gentle* physical therapy or neuromuscular re-education (*e.g. Trager therapy, See Appendix K*) can be very helpful. A recent pilot study giving lidocaine 240 mg IV over 40 minutes (with patients on a monitor) once a week for four weeks resulted in marked improvement in eight of eleven patients.[30]

Anxiety and depression. CFIDS patients are often appropriately depressed and/or anxious over their disability. Studies show that the depression is usually caused by the illness and the illness is *not* caused by depression.[31] This is true with any disabling illness. Antidepressants often help. Using Prozac, Zoloft, or Paxil can often improve the patient's quality of life. Start with a low dose (e.g. Prozac 10 mg) and slowly increase as needed. Desyrel can often help with anxiety and is also not addictive.

Coenzyme Q10. 30-50 mg three times a day (OTC) is sometimes helpful (it may take four to five weeks to see the effect).

Evening primrose oil *(500 mg)*. Two capsules four times a day plus MAX EPA (Fish oil) 1000 mg/d is sometimes helpful (OTC—it takes three months to see full effect).

Treat nasal congestion *(See Table 14-5)*.

Gamma globulin. Consider an empiric trial of gammar (gamma globulin) 4-5 cc IM weekly for five weeks if recurrent infections or severe fatigue persists.

Magnesium sulfate. If mg < 1.6, consider 2 gram IM q. week for four weeks (add lidocaine 2 percent .1 cc to decrease soreness from the shot). Give 2 cc of 50 percent solution (1 gm) in each buttock (do *not* use 50 percent solution IV!) and have the patient wait in the office for 30 minutes (if dizziness occurs, have patient lay down until it passes).

Calcium with Vitamin D *(1000-1500 mg/d)*. If Fibromyalgia persists.

When all else fails Dr. Jay Goldstein has added new tools. Dr. Goldstein is a Los Angeles physician who is a leading research expert on the role of neurotransmitters and CNS dysfunctions in CFS. In his upcoming book *Treatment Options in CFS* (to be published by Haworth Press in 1995),[32] he discusses medications that often help CFS patients. Whether or not a medication will help an individual patient should be apparent within one hour of the first dose. Because of this, empirically trying one dose of each medication each hour (one at a time) during symptomatic days is a reasonable approach. Stop when you find the one that works. This is best done in your office under supervision (CFS patients are often subject to medication side effects). Among his many recommendations are:

1. Felbatol (Felbamate) 400 mg t.i.d.—A NMDA receptor antagonistic, (potentially toxic).
2. Cognex 10 mg t.i.d. or q.i.d.—This is a centrally acting cholinesterase inhibitor. You need to monitor liver function tests weekly if on cognex.
3. Nimodipine—A calcium channel antagonist. Dr. Goldstein feels this is the most beneficial medication he currently uses.
4. Risperdal (Risperidone)—A serotonin ($5-HT_2$) receptor antagonist. At high doses, it is also a dopamine (D2) receptor antagonist that is helpful in schizo-

phrenia. Use very low doses (.25-1 mg b.i.d.).

5. Oxytocin—10 units p.o. q.d. (via Belmar Pharmacy). This is also a hypothalamic neurotransmittor[33] and is worth trying in patients with pallor and cold extremities. Begin after the patient's DHEA has been normalized for three months. Dr. Jorge Flechas (another CFS researcher) has found this to be very useful. It takes less than two weeks to see the effect.

6. Calan 60-120 mg q.h.s.

7. See Appendix M for more of Dr. Goldstein's recommendations. Although this multi-dimensional approach takes some time and practice to learn, I suspect you will find it very helpful in treating your chronic fatigue patients. I would recommend reading his book before using his protocol. I would also recommend reading my study (See Appendix A) and the rest of this book as time goes on. For those of you who would like more depth, I've listed some excellent books in a short list of recommended reading (See Appendix L). I think you will find it as exciting as I have to watch your CFS and Fibromyalgia patients turn vibrant!

Table 14-1

**A CASE OF THE CHRONIC FATIGUE SYNDROME
IS DEFINED BY THE PRESENCE OF THE FOLLOWING:**

1. Clinically evaluated, unexplained, persistent, or relapsing chronic fatigue that is of new or definite onset (has not been lifelong); is not the result of ongoing exertion; is not substantially alleviated by rest; and results in substantial reduction in previous levels of occupational, educational, social, or personal activities.

2. Concurrent occurrence of four or more of the following symptoms, all of which must have persisted or recurred during six or more consecutive months of illness and must not have predated the fatigue:

   A. Self-reported impairment in short-term memory or concentration severe enough to cause substantial reduction in previous levels of occupational, educational, social, or personal activities.

   B. Sore throat.

   C. Tender cervical or axillary lymph nodes.

   D. Muscle pain.

   E. Multijoint pain without joint swelling or redness.

   F. Headaches of a new type, pattern, or severity.

   G. Unrefreshing sleep.

   H. Postexertional malaise lasting more than 24 hours.

14 December 94, Annals of Internal Medicine, *Volume 121, Number 12*

Table 14-2

RECOMMENDED LAB TESTS

Most Important	Helpful (as needed in each patient)
1. Total T3, Free T4, TSH	1. Thyroid antibodies (especially with Fibromyalgia)
2. Chem 19	2. Lymes titer (if common in your area)
3. CBC with diff.	3. RPR
4. ESR	4. Latex fixation
5. Magnesium	5. HgbA1C
6. Fe, TIBC, ferritin	6. IgE
7. U/A with micro	7. FSH and LH
8. ANA.	8. Stool C. difficile
9. B-12 level.	9. Allergy testing
10. Stool O&P, Giardia and Cryptosporidium and quantitative yeast (must be done in a lab *specializing* in parasitology—otherwise they will miss most parasites). Can be done in our lab by mail *(See Appendix N)*	10. Sleep testing (if male or if overweight, or if sleep apnea or restless leg syndrome are suspected)
11. CPK.	11. Sinus CT (if sinusitis persists despite treatment)
12. HIV	12. C-reactive protein
13. Cortrosyn stimulation test.	13. PPD
14. Yeast questionnaire *(See Appendix C)*	14. Elimination diet (and/or blood tests) if needed (for food sensitivities)
15. DHEA level	15. Testosterone levels
16. Stool and/or serum ameba antibodies	

If desired, the blood and stool tests (except for the cortrosyn test) can be done by mail in our office. Treatment recommendations will then be sent based on the test results (See Appendix N).

Table 14-3

TESTS THAT NEED TO BE INTERPRETED DIFFERENTLY IN CFIDS AND FIBROMYALGIA (BECAUSE OF HYPOTHALAMIC AND IMMUNE DYSFUNCTION)

Thyroid testing. Recheck TSH, T3 and T4 six weeks after changing medication.

1. Total T3—if low normal, consider a trial of Armour thyroid ¼-1 grain each morning.

2. Free T4—If low normal, consider a trial of Synthroid 25 mcg 1-3 tablets each a.m. If the patient feels worse on the treatment, this may indicate adrenal insufficiency (or patient was euthyroid). If no change, consider changing to Armour thyroid ½-1 grain q.a.m.

3. TSH—If over 3.5 or under .9 (with a low normal Free T3 or T4) consider treatment as above.

4. Thyroid antibodies—If positive, consider a trial of Synthroid, 25-75 mcg q.a.m. (unless T4 is high or high normal—in which case hyperthyroidism may be contributing to the fatigue).

Cortrosyn stimulation testing. If the baseline cortisol is < 12 mcg/dl or if the cortisol level doesn't double at one hour (and is < 40 mcg/dl) consider a trial of cortef 5 mg t.i.d. with meals. The cortef can be adjusted up to 30 mg/d. Review the controversial nature of the treatment with the patient. If the patient is not diabetic or hypertensive, the main risk at this dose is gastritis. Add calcium with Vitamin D if the patient is taking over 15 mg of cortef per day.

Magnesium. I treat all fatigue patients with magnesium chloride or lactate 67 mg or Ultra Malic (magnesium plus malic acid—available through CFIDS Buyer's Club) two tablets three times a day for eight months. Then take two tablets a day. If the magnesium level is < 1.8, this is very suggestive of low magnesium stores. Use less magnesium if diarrhea occurs, or if the creatinine is elevated.

B-12 level. I recommend a trial of B-12 1 mg IM weekly for eight to ten weeks if the B-12 level is < 540 pg/ml or if the patient does not respond to other treatments. If the patient improves but the effect wears off, continue 1 mg IM every one to four weeks as needed.

Stool tests. I treat all parasites. If yeast overgrowth (1+ or greater) is present or if the yeast questionnaire (*See Appendix C*) is positive, I treat with Nystatin and Sporanox or Diflucan.

Iron studies. If the percent saturation is < 20 or ferritin is < 40 mg/l, treat with iron. Chromagen or Ferrous Sequels, one twice a day are less constipating than some others. If not tolerated, "herbal iron formulas" (at health food stores) are helpful. Do not give iron within four hours of thyroid medication or the thyroid will *not* be absorbed!

DHEA. If low (< 150 mcg/dl) consider a trial of DHEA 5-50 mg p.o. q.d. to bring the DHEA level to within 150-250 mcg/dl. DHEA can be ordered by telephone (Professional Arts Pharmacy (800) 832-9285 or Belmar Pharmacy (800) 525-9473).

Table 14-4

RECOMMENDED TREATMENT

1. TwinLab Daily One caps or Berocca Plus multivitamin (one a day).
2. Magnesium malate *(See Appendix K),* chloride, or lactate (Slow-Mag or Mag-Tabs SR) two tablets three times a day for eight months, then two a day (less if diarrhea).
3. No sweets, alcohol, or caffeine for three to six months (expect withdrawal symptoms the first week). Then limit these to moderate amounts.
4. Sleep at least eight hours a night.
5. Slowly begin an exercise program as the patient improves.
6. Treat with Synthroid or Armour thyroid if symptoms suggest hypothyroidism (even if tests are normal).
7. Treat low or borderline adrenal function (with cortef and/or DHEA). Try Florinef .1 mg p.o. q.d. if patient is hypotensive. (Monitor for hypokalemia).
8. Consider treatment with estrogen in females or testosterone in males if these are low.
9. Treat any bowel infections.
10. Treat any yeast overgrowth. Avoid antibiotics when possible.
11. Treat any sinusitis and/or nasal congestion.
12. Consider vitamin B-12 1 mg IM q. week for eight to ten weeks then p.r.n.
13. If Fibromyalgia: Use low-dose Elavil, Desyrel, Flexeril, Ambien, Soma, or herbals for sleep.
14. If anxiety—consider Desyrel.
15. If depression or frustration—consider Paxil, Prozac, or Zoloft. These may help even in the absence of depression.
16. Counseling to uncover life conflicts, etc. (I recommend Jungian).
17. If Fibromyalgia persists, consider SL NTG, p.o. calcium, and/or Klonopin.
18. If fatigue persists, consider Coenzyme Q10, evening primrose oil with Max EPA, IM magnesium, IM gamma globulin.
19. See Appendix M for Dr. Jay Goldstein's treatment protocol.

Table 14-5

NASAL CONGESTION/SINUSITIS THERAPY

Dr. Chester recommends trying the following therapeutic trial for nasal congestion/sinusitis:

1. Keflex (500 mg four times a day) for one week followed by doxycycline (100 mg two times a day) for one week if there is no improvement (prescription antibiotics).

2. Xylometazoline 0.1 percent nasal spray three times a day for three days (prescription).

3. Sudafed 60 mg, four times a day or 120 mg (sustained release) two times a day (may cause shakiness or palpitations).

4. Nasal steam inhalations, 20 minutes three times a day.

5. Sleep eight hours a night.

6. No beer, wine, or milk products.

Table 14-6A

NORMAL DHEA LEVELS (MCG/DL)

	Age Group	5th Percentile	50th Percentile	95th Percentile
	10-19	—	140	—
	20-29	65	185	380
	30-39	45	150	270
Females	40-49	32	120	240
	50-59	26	85	200
	60-69	13	50	130
	70-79	17	40	90
	80-89	—	26	—
	Postmenopausal	10	55	190
	10-19	—	215	—
	20-29	280	420	640
	30-39	120	300	520
Males	40-49	95	250	530
	50-59	70	160	310
	60-69	42	130	290
	70-79	28	80	175
	80-89	—	36	—

Many workers in this area recommend keeping everyone's DHEA at least 150 mcg/dl (See Table 14 B and C) and at least at the 50th percentile. If acne or hirsutism (in females—facial hair growth) occurs, decrease the dose.

Table 14-6B

AGE-ADJUSTED 12-YEAR MORTALITY RATES
IN MEN AGED 50 TO 79 YEARS, ACCORDING TO DHEA-S CATEGORY

DHEAS Category	No of Subjects	All Causes	Cause of Death		
			Cardiovascular Disease	Ischemic Heart Disease	Cancer
				rate per 100 men	
All subjects					
DHEAS <140 mcg/dl	132	35.5	20.3	16.4	7.1
DHEAS >140 mcg/dl	110	26.6	8.3	7.5	6.2
Relative risk		1.3	2.4*	2.2	1.1
Men with no history of heart disease at the base line					
DHEAS<140 mcg/dl	108	38.5	20.9	16.8	8.3
DHEAS>140 mcg/dl	100	26.0	6.4	5.3	6.5
Relative risk		1.5	3.3*	3.2*	1.3
All subjects except those who died within 2 yr					
DHEAS<140 mcg/dl	125	33.3	19.7	15.3	6.4
DHEAS>140 mcg/dl	108	24.9	7.3	6.4	5.0
Relative risk		1.3	2.7*	2.5*	1.3
All subjects, according to tertile					
DHEAS<110 mcg/dl	88	34.2	20.4	14.4	6.1
DHEAS>110<180 mcg/dl	75	37.6	15.0	13.9	11.0
DHEAS>180 mcg/dl	79	22.1	6.8	6.8	7.4

*$P<0.05$

Table 14-6C

MEAN BASE-LINE DHEAS LEVELS, ACCORDING TO 12-YEAR MORTALITY RATES, IN MEN AGED 50 TO 79 YEARS*

Age Group	All Causes		Cardiovascular Disease		Ischemic Heart Disease	
	Alive (N=166)	Dead (N=76)	Non-CVD[1] (N=204) µg/dl	CVD (N=38)	Non-IHD[2] (N=211)	IHD (N=31)
All subjects						
50-54	277±146	102±0	277±146	102±0	277±146	102±0
55-59	213±112	129±7	210±111	124±0	210± 111	124±0
60-64	157±79	136±44	155±76	135±52	155±76	135±52
65-69	156±78	114±48	147±75	112±45	142±75	137±33
70-74	136±94	120±62	135±83	104±55	132±81	107±62
75-79	100±35	79±43	91±83	71±24	93±47	71±24
Total	180±110	114±54	169±105	107±49	166±104	111±51
Age-Adjusted	168	141	164	131	163	135
Mean	P=0.048		P=0.039		P=0.119	

Men with no history of heart disease at base line

	(N=143)	(N=65)	(N=178)	(N=30)	(N=184)	(N=24)
50-54	273±133	102±0	273±133	102±0	273±133	102±0
55-59	226±114	129±7	223±113	124±0	223±113	124±0
60-64	172±79	133±46	170±77	135±52	170±77	135±52
65-69	161±77	110±45	150±74	103±37	145±74	124±21
70-74	143±97	128±62	141±85	108±57	139±83	113±65
75-79	100±35	84±47	99±45	68±28	99±46	68±28
Total	186±107	117±53	174±102	108±48	171±101	114±50
Age-Adjusted	176	140	171	126	169	131
Mean	P=0.014		P=0.010		P=0.046	

*P values refer to comparisons between groups, and plus-minus values are mean±SD.

[1] Non-CVD refers to all living subjects and all subjects who did not die of cardiovascular disease during the 12-year follow-up period. CVD refers to all subjects who died of cardiovascular disease (including ischemic heart disease) during the 12-year follow-up period.

[2] Non-IHD refers to all living subjects and all subjects who did not die of ischemic heart disease during the 12-year follow-up period. IHD refers to all subjects who died of ischemic heart disease during the 12-year follow-up period.

From Barrett-Connor E, Khaw KT, Yen SSC: A prospective study of dehydroepiandrosterone sulfate, mortality, and cardiovascular diseaes. N Engl J Med 315:1519-1524, 1986; Table 14-6B.

References/Bibliography

INTRODUCTION

1. Teitelbaum, J., & Bird, B. Effective Treatment of Severe Chronic Fatigue States. *J. Musculoskeletal Pain* (1995): Issue 4.

CHAPTER 1

1. Holmes, G.P., Kaplan, J.E., et al. Chronic Fatigue Syndrome: A Working Case Definition. *Annals of Internal Medicine* (1988): 108, 3: 387-9.
2. Bell, D.S., & Donev, S. *Curing Fatigue*. Emmaus, PA.: Rodale Press, 1993.
3. Price, R.K., North, C.S., et al. Estimating the Presence of CFS in the Community. *Public Health Reports* (Sept-Oct 1992): 107: 514-22.
4. Marchesani, R.B. Critical Antiviral Pathway Deficient in CFS Patients. *Infectious Disease News* (August 1993): 4.
5. Goldenberg, D.L. Fibromyalgia Syndrome. *JAMA* (1987): 257: 2782-87.
6. Strauss, S.E., Fritz, S., Dale, J.K., Gould, B., & Strober, W. Lymphocyte Phenotype and Function in CFS. *J Clin Immun* (Jan 1993): 13; 30-40.
7. Teitelbaum, J., & Bird, B. Effective Treatment of Severe Chronic Fatigue States. *J. Musculoskeletal Pain* (1995): Issue 4.
8. Halpin, D, & Wessely, S. VP-1 Antigen in Chronic Postviral Fatigue Syndrome. *Lancet* (1989): 1: 1028-9.
9. Yousef, G.E., Bell, E.J., et al. Chronic Enterovirus Infection in Patients with

Postviral Fatigue Syndrome. *Lancet* (1988): 1: 146-7.

10. Archard, L.E., Bowles, N.E., Behan, P.O., et al. Postviral Fatigue Syndrome Persistence of Enterovirus RNA in Muscle and Elevated Creatine Kinase. *Journal of the Royal Society of Medicine* (1988): 81: 326-9.

11. Wakefield, D., Lloyd, A., & Dwyer, J.. Human Herpes Virus 6 and Myalgic Encephalomyelitis. *Lancet* (1988): 1: 1059.

12. Jeffries, W. *Safe Uses of Cortisone*. Springfield, IL: Charles C. Thomas, 1981.

13. Hyde, B.M. *The Clinical and Scientific Basis of M.E./CFS*. Ottawa,Ontario: Nightingale Research Foundation, 1992.

14. Neeck, G., & Riedel, W. Thyroid Function in Patients with Fibromyalgia Syndrome. *Journal of Rheumatology* (1992): 19: 1120-2.

15. Demitrack, M.A., Dale, J.K., Strauss, S.E., et al. Evidence for Impaired Activation of the Hypothalamic-Pituitary-Adrenal Axis in Patients with CFS. *J Clin Endo Metab* (1991): 73: 1223-34.

16. McCain, G.A., & Tilbe, K.S. Diurnal Hormone Variation in Fibromyalgia Syndrome. *Journal of Rheumatology* (1993): 25: 469-474.

17. Bakheit, A.M.O., Behan, P.O., Dinan, T.G., et al. Possible Up Regulation of Hypothalamic 5-HT Receptors in Patients With Postviral Fatigue Syndrome. *BMJ* (April 1992): 304: 1010-12.

18. Griep, E.N., Boersma, J.N., et al. Altered Reactivity of the HPA Axis in the Primary Fibromyalgia Syndrome. *Journal of Rheumatology* (1993): 20: 469-474.

117

CHAPTER 2

1. Marston, R.M., & Peterkin, B.B. Nutrient Content of the National Food Supply. *National Food Review* (Winter 1980): 21-25.

2. Nelson, J.H. Wheat—Its Processing and Utilization. *Am J Clin Nutr* (May 1985): 41;#5 (suppl.): 1070-6.

3. Schroeder, H.A. Loss of Vitamins and Trace Minerals Resulting From Processing and Preservation of Foods. *Am J Clin Nutr* (May 1971): 24: 562-73.

4. Eaton, S.B. Paleolithic Nutrition. *NEJM* (Jan. 31, 1985): 312 #5: 283-9.

5. Trowell, H.C. (Ed). *Western Diseases: Their Emergence and Prevention*. Cambridge, Mass: Harvard University Press, 1981.

6. Mertz, W. (Ed). Beltsville One Year Dietary Intake Survey. *Am J Clin Nutr*

(Dec 1984): 40 (supp.): 1323-1403.

7. Crook, W. *The Yeast Connection and the Woman,* Jackson, Tennessee: Professional Books, 1995.

CHAPTER 3

1. Travell, J.G., & Simons, D.G. *Myofascial Pain and Dysfunction: The Trigger Point Manual, Vol 1.* Baltimore, MD.: Williams & Wilkins: 4-Perpetuating Factors: 103-164 (excellent chapter with 317 references—saved me from getting writers cramp from having to list them!—See Appendix B for a summary).

2. Kennes, B., et al. *Gerontology* (1983): 29(5); 305-10.

3. Chandra, R.K. Effect of Macro and Micro Nutrient Deficiencies and Excesses on Immune Response. *Food Technology* (Feb 1985): 91-3.

4. Chandra, S., et al. Undernutrition Impairs Immunity. *Internal Medicine* (Dec 1984): 5, #13.; 85-99.

5. Chandra, R.K., et al. NIH workshop on Trace Element Regulation of Immunity and Infection. *Nutrition Research* (1982): 2: 721-733.

6. Talbott, M.C. *Am J Clin Nutr* (1987): 46: 659-664.

7. Moydan, S.K., et al. *Am J Clin Nutr* (1990): 52: 557-563. (There are hundreds/thousands of references on the importance of vitamins and minerals on immune function. If you have a lot of free time, run a Medline computer search on immune function and various vitamins and minerals.)

8. Seelig, M.S. The Requirement of Magnesium by the Normal Adult. *Am J Clin Nutr* (June 1964): 14: 342-390 (177 references).

9. Lakshmanad, F.L., et al. Magnesium Intakes and Balances. *Am J Clin Nutr* (Dec.1984): 40(supp):1380-9.

10. Hoes, M.J. *ACTA Psychiat Belg.* (1981): 81: 72-4.

11. Harrisons. *Principles of Internal Medicine*, 11th Edition: 1496.

12. Walter, T., et al. *Am J Clin Nutr* (1986): 44: 877-882.

13. *JAMA* (8/5/88): 260, #5: 607.

14. Darnell, L.S. *Am J Clin Nutr* (Supplement 31st Annual ASCN meeting). Abstract 21.

15. Rushton, D.C., et al. *Lancet* (June 22): 1991; 1554.

16. Lindenbaum, J., Healton, E.B., et al. Neuropsychiatric Disorders Caused by

Cobalamin Deficiency in the Absence of Anemia or Macrocytoses. *NEJM* (1988): 318: 1720-8.

17. NEJM Editorial on B-12 *NEJM* (1988): 318.

18. Lindenbaum, J., et al. Prevalence of Cobalamin Deficiency in the Framingham Elderly Population. *Am J Clin Nutr* (1994): 60: 2-11.

19. Karnaze, D.S., et al. *Arch Int Med* (1987): 147: 429-31.

20. Carethers, M. *Geriatrics* (March 1988): 43, #3: 89-112.

21. Herbert, V. Editorial. *Arch Int Med* (Aug 1988): 148: 1705

22. Allen, H.A., & Casterline, J. *Am J Clin Nutr* (1994): 60: 12-14.

CHAPTER 4

1. Teitelbaum, J., & Bird, B. Effective Treatment of Severe Chronic Fatigue States. *J. Musculoskeletal Pain* (1995): Issue 4.

2. Jeffries, W.M. *Safe uses of Cortisone.* Springfield, IL: Charles C. Thomas, 1981.

3. Personal Communication.

4. Anderson, R.A., et al. Chromium & Hypoglycemia. *Am J Clin Nutr* (April 1985): 41, #4; 841.

5. Jeffries, W. Low Dose Glucocorticoid Therapy. *Archives of Int. Med* (1967): 119: 265-278.

6. Zellssen, P.M.J., et al. *Annals of Internal Medicine* (1994): 120: 207-210.

7. Meikle, A.W., Daynes, R.A., & Araned, B.A., Adrenal Androgen Secretion & Biologic Effects. *End/Metab Clinics of N. America.* (June 1991): 20,#2: 381-400.

8. Parker, L.N. Control of Adrenal Androgen Secretion. IBID: 401-421.

9. Barrett-Connor, E., Khaw, R.T., & Yen, S.C. A Prospective Study of DHEA, Mortality & Cardiovascular Disease. *NEJM* (1986): 315: 1519-1524.

10. Rowe, P.C., Bole-Hoiaighah, I., Kan, J.S., & Calkins, H. Is Neurally Mediated Hypotension an Unrecognized Cause of Chronic Fatigue? *Lancet* (March 11, 1995): 345: 623-4.

CHAPTER 5

1. Faglia, G., et al. Thyrotropin Secretion in Patients with Central Hypothyroidism. *J Clin Endocrinol Metab* (1979): 48: 989-998.

2. Teitelbaum, J., & Bird, B. *Effective Treatment of Chronic Fatigue States.* (1995).

3. Travell, J.G., & Simons, D.G. *Myofascial Pain & Dysfunction: The Trigger Point Manual, Vol 1.* Baltimore, MD.: Williams & Wilkins: 4 Perpetuating Factors: 103-164

4. Sorkin, L.S. *Head, Neck, TMJ Pain & Dysfunction*, Philadelphia: Saunders, 1977: 140-180.

5. Travell, J. *Arch Phys Med Rehab.* (1981): 62: 100-106.

6. Simons, D.G. *Myofascial Pain Syndrome Due to Trigger Points*; Int Rehab Med Assn Monograph Series #1: Nov. 1987.

CHAPTER 6

1. Alexander, W. *Int Med World Report* (Jan 1-14, 1995): 32.

2. Gambrell, R.D. *Consultant* (July 1994): 1047-1057.

3. Brock, M. *ACTA Neurochirurgical* (suppl)(1990): 47, 127-8 .

4. Jenkins, J.S. The Role of Oxytocin: Present Concepts. *Clinical Endocrinology* (1991): 34: 515-25.

5. Personal Communication—Jorge Flechas, M.D. and JS Jenkins.

CHAPTER 7

1. Vance, M.L. Hypopituitarism. *NEJM:* 330, #23: 1651-62.

2. McGauley, G.A. Quality of Life Assessment Before & After Growth Hormone Treatment in Adults with GH deficiency. *Acta Pediatr Scand* (Suppl) (1989): 356: 70-2.

3. Cuneo, R.C., Salomen, F., et al. GH Treatment in Growth Hormone Deficient Adults II. Effects on Exercise Performance. *J Appl Physiol* (1991): 70: 695-700.

4. Jorgensen, J.O.L., Pedersen, S.A., et al. Long Term GH Treatment in Growth Hormone Deficient Adults. *ACTA Endocrinol* (1991): 125: 449-453.

5. Bennet, R.B., Clark, S.R., et al. Low Levels of Somatomedin C in Patients With the Fibromyalgia Syndrome. *Arth Rheum* (1992): 35: 1113-6.

6. Bakheit, A.M.O., Behan, P.O., et al. Abnormal Anginine-vasopression Secretion & Water Metabolism in Patients with Post-Viral Fatigue Syndrome. *ACTA Neurol Scand* (1993): 87: 234-8.

CHAPTER 8

1. Quesada, J.R., Talpaz, M., et al. Clinical Toxicity of Interferon in Cancer Patients: A review. *J. Clin Oncology* (Feb 1986): 4: 234-43.

2. Adams, F., Avesada, J.R., et al. Neuropsychiatric Manifestations of Human Leukocyte Interferon Therapy in Patients with Cancer. *JAMA* (1984): 252: 938-41.

3. Meikle, A.W., Parker, L,N,, et al. *Endo and Metab Clinics of North America* (June 1991): 381-421.

4. Barker, E., Fujimura, S..F, et al. Immunologic Abnormalities Associated with CFS. *Clin Infectious Dis* (1994): 18 (suppl 1): 5136-41.

5. Aoki, T., Miyakoshi, H., et al. Low NK Syndrome and Its Relationship to CFS. *Clin Immunol and Immunopath* (Dec 1993): 69, #3: 253-65.

CHAPTER 9

1. Crook, W., *The Yeast Connection and the Woman*. Jackson, Tennessee: Professional Books,1995.

2. Pochant, P. *Am J Clin Nutr* (Jan 1992): 55: 78-80.

3. Reid, G. *Lancet* (Oct 29, 1994): 344: 1229.

4. Edman, J., et al. *Am J Obstet and Gynecol* (1986): 155: 1082-8.

5. Boyne, R. *J Nutr* (1982): 116(5): 816-822.

6. Inhouse research data available through Proctor and Gamble.

7. Avorn, J. *JAMA* (1994): 271: 751-754.

CHAPTER 10

1. Deckelbaum, R.J. ELISA More Accurate than Microscopy for Giardia: *Infectious Diseases in Children* (Oct 1993): 30.

2. Holmes, G.P., et al: *Ann Intern Med* (1988): 108, #3: 387-9.

3. Galland, L., et al: Giardia as a Cause of Chronic Fatigue. *J Nutr Med* (1990): 2-031.

4. Gittleman, A.L., *Guess What Came to Dinner—Parasites and Your Health*: Garden City Park, NJ: Avery Publishing, 1993.

5. Simons, D.G. *Myofascial Pain Syndrome Due to Trigger Points*: Int Rehab Med Assn Monograph Series #1, Nov 1987.

6. Travell, J.G., & Simons, D.G. *Myofascial Pain and Dysfunction: The Trigger Point Manual Vol 1*: Baltimore, MD: Williams & Wilkins: 103-164.

CHAPTER 11

1. Travell, J.G., & Simons, D.G. *Myofascial Pain and Dysfunction: The Trigger Point Manual Vol 1*: Baltimore, MD: Williams & Wilkins: 103-164.
2. McCain, G.A., Tilbe KS. Diurnal Hormone Variation in Fibromyalgia Syndrome. *J Rheumatol* (1993): 25: 469-474.
3. Neeck, G., & Riedel, W. Thyroid Function in Patients With Fibromyalgia Syndrome. *J Rheumatol* (1992): 19: 1120-22
4. Moldofsky, H. *Sleep and CFS in CFS*, Dawson, D. & Sabin, S. (ed). Boston: Little, Brown and Company, 1993: 10.
5. Bennett, R.M., Gatter, R.A., et al. Cyclobenzaprine versus Placebo in Fibromyalgia: Arthritis and Rheumatism (Dec 1988): 31, #12:1535-42.
6. Gatter, R.A. Pharmacotherapeutics in Fibromyalgia. *Am J Med* (Sept 29,1986): 81(sup 3A):63-66.
7. Dressing, H., & Riemann, D. Insomnia. Are Valerian/Melissa Combinations of equal value to Benzodiazepine? *Therapiewoche* (1992): 42: 726-736.
8. Personal Communication—Jay Goldstein, M.D.

CHAPTER 12

1. Strosberg, J. *Rheumatology for the Practicing Physician*. (Jan 1989): 12.
2. Smythe, H. IBID: 13-14.
3. Griep, E.N., Boersma, J., et al. *J Rheumatol* (1993): 20: 469-474.

CHAPTER 13

1. Forman, PhD, R.; *How to Control Your Allergies*. Atlanta: Larchmont Books: 1979.
2. Rogers, S. *Tired or Toxic*. Syracuse: Prestige Publishing, 1990.
3. Rogers, S. Chemical Sensitivity—Breaking the Paralyzing Paradigm, Part I. *Int Med World Report* (1992): 7, #3: 1.
4. IBID. Part II (1992): 7, #6: 8, 21-31.
5. Chester, A.C. *Chronic Fatigue of Nasal Origin: Possible Confusion with CFS in The Clinical and scientific Basis of ME/CFS*. Hyde BM (ed). Ottawa, Ontario:

Nightingale Foundation, 1992: 260-266.

6. May, K.P., West, S.G., et al. Sleep Apnea in Male Patients with Fibromyalgia: *Am J Med* (May 1993): 94: 505-8.

7. John Hopkins Medical Letter. (Oct 1994): 5-6 (for info send SASE to Restless Leg Foundation, P.O. Box 314-JH, 514 Daniels St., Raleigh, NC 27605.)

8. Thompson, C., Stanson, D., Smith, A. *Lancet* (1990): 336: 703-6.

9. Rosenthal, N., Diagnosis and Treatment of Seasonal Affective Disorder; *JAMA*. (in press).

10. Liebermann, J., Bell, D.S. *Am J. Med* (1993): 95: 407-412.

11. O'Rourke, et al. Treatment of Seasonal Depression with d-Fenluramine *J Clin Psychiatry* (1989). 50: 343-7.

12. Ruhrmann, S., & Kasper, S. Seasonal Depression. *Medizinische Monatsschrift TUR Pharmazeuten* (1992): 15; 293-9.

13. Ft. Lauderdale CFIDS Conference, (Oct 7-9, 1994).

14. Goldstein, J. Fibromyalgia. *Clinical Rheumatology* (Nov 94): 8, #4: ch 5.

CHAPTER 14

1. Sternberg, E.M. Hypoimmune Fatigue Syndromes. Disease of the Stress Response. *J Rheumatol* (1993): 20: 418-21.

2. Neeck, G., & Riedel, W. Thyroid function in Patients with Fibromyalgia Syndrome. *J Rheumatol* (1992): 19: 1120-2.

3. Demitrack, M.A., et al. Evidence for Impaired Activation of the Hypothalamic-Pituitary-Adrenal Axis in Patients with CFS. *J Clin Endo Metab* (1991): 73: 1224-34.

4. Bakheit, A.M.O., & Behan, P.O. Possible Upregulation of Hypothalamic 5HT Receptors in Patients with Postviral Fatigue Syndrome. *BMJ* (April 1992): 304: 1010-2.

5. Griep, E.N., et al. Altered Reactivity of the HPA Axis in the Primary Fibromyalgia Syndrome. *J Rheumatol* (1993): 20: 469-474.

6. McCain, G.A., & Tilbe, K.S. Diurnal Hormone Variation in Fibromyalgia Syndrome and a Comparison With Rheumatoid Arthritis. *J Rheumatol* (1993): 25: 469-474.

7. Crook, W. *The Yeast Connection*, Jackson, Tennessee: Professional Books, 1983.

8. Galland, L., et al: Giardia as Cause of Chronic Fatigue. *J Nutr Med* (1990): 27-31.

9. Travell, J.G., & Simons, D.G. *Myofascial Pain and Dysfunction: The Trigger point Manual, Vol 1*: Baltimore, MD: Williams & Wilkins,1983; 103-164.

10. Chandra, R.K. Effect of Macro and Micro Nutrient Deficiencies and Excess on Immune Response. *Food Technology* (Feb 1985): 91-93.

11. Chandra, R.K., et al. NIH Workshop on Trace Element Regulation of Immunity and Infection. *Nutr Research* (1982): 2: 721-733.

12. Chandra, S., et al. Undernutrition Impaired Immunity. *Internal Medicine* (Dec 1984): 5, #13: 85-99.

13. Talbott, M.C. *Am J Clin Nutr* (1987): 46: 659-664.

14. Moydan, S., et al. *Am J Clin Nutr* (1990): 52: 557-563. (These are just a few. Reading the chapter in reference 9 above and A Medline of Different Nutrients and Immunity will likely supply over 1000 references.)

15. Chester, A.C. *Chronic Fatigue of Nasal Origin*. In the Clinical Basis of CFS/ME. Hyde, BM (ed). Ottawa, Ontario: Nightingale Foundation, 1992: 260-266.

16. Faglia, G., et al. Thyrotropin Secretion in Patients with Central Hypothyroidism. *J Clin Endocrinol Metab* (1979): 48: 989-998.

17. Campbell, N.R., et al. *Annals of Internal Medicine* (1992): 117: 1010-1013.

18a. Hoes, M.J. *ACTA Psychiatr Belg* (1981): 81: 72-4.

18b. Dykner, J. *Am Heart J.* (Jan 1979).

19. Abraham, G.E., & Flechas, J. Management of Fibromyalgia: Rationale for the Use of Magnesium and Malic Acid. *J of Nutritional Medicine* (1992): 3: 49-59.

20. Rushton, D.H., et al. *Lancet* (June 22, 1991): 1554.

20b. Kirn, T.F. *JAMA* (8/5/88): 607.

21. Lindenbaum, J., et al. Neuropsychiatric Disorders Caused by Cobalamin deficiency in the Absence of Anemia in Macrocytosis. *NEJM* (1988): 318: 1720-28.

22. Lindenbaum, J, et al. Prevalence of Cobalamin Deficiency in the Framingham Elderly Population. *Am J Clin Nutr* (1994): 60: 2-11.

23. Norman, E.J. *Am J Med* (June 93): 94: 589-594.

24. Deckelbaum, R.J.. ELISA More Accurate Than O&P for Giardia. *Infectious Diseases in Children* (Oct 1993): 30.

25. Personal Communication—W. Jeffries.

26. Jeffries, W. *Safe Uses of Cortisol*. Springfield, IL:Charles C. Thomas, 1981.

27. Jeffries, W. Low Dose Glucocorticoid Therapy. *Archives of Internal Medicine* (1967): 119: 265-278.

28. Barrett-Connor, E., Khaw, K.T., & Yen, S.S.C. A Prospective Study of DHEA-S, Mortality, and Cardiovascular Disease. *NEJM* (1986): 315: 1519-1524.

29. Morales, A.J., et al. Effects of DHEA in Advancing Age. *J. Clin Endo Metab* (1994): 78: 1360-7.

30. Posner, I.A. Treatment of Fibromyalgia Syndrome with IV Lidocaine: A Prospective, Randomized Pilot Study. *J. Musculoskeletal Pain* (1994): 2(4): 55-65.

31. Griep, E.N., et al. Altered Reactivity of the HPA Axis in the Primary Fibromyalgia Syndrome. *J. Rheumatol* (1993): 20: 469-474.

32. Goldstein, J. *The CFIDS Chronicle* (Summer 1994): 82-6.

33. Brock, M., *ACTA Neurochirurgica* (suppl) (1990): 47, 127-8.

Appendix A

Study on Effective Treatment of Severe Chronic Fatigue States

Unfortunately, we have found that we cannot print the study until it is published later in 1995 in the *Journal of Musculoskeletal Pain* (Issue 4, Winter 1995). If you would like a copy (after November 1995) please send a self-addressed, stamped envelope (large envelope with two stamps) to:

Jacob Teitelbaum, M.D.
139 Old Solomons Island Road
Annapolis, MD 21401

Appendix B

Perpetuating Factors in Myofascial Pain

By David Simons, M.D.

Perpetuating Factors

The presence or absence of perpetuating factors determines the answer to the question, "How long should the effect of specific myofascial therapy last?" In the absence of perpetuating factors, relief should last indefinitely until the TP* is reactivated, as in the beginning, by another over-load stress. In the presence of perpetuating factors, relief is temporary; lasting relief depends on eliminating perpetuating factors [36,42] so that the effect of successive therapy is cumulative.

In a few patients, the muscles become so hyperirritable due to perpetuating factors that any attempt at specific myofascial therapy aggravates the pain. The perpetuating factors must be addressed first. In severe cases, perpetuating factors are usually multiple.

A significant perpetuating factor may have caused no symptoms before activation of the TPs. A leg length discrepancy of 6 mm (¼") may have caused no pain or discomfort throughout most of a lifetime; upon activation of quadratus lumborum TPs by another stress, the discrepancy becomes a potent perpetuator of those TPs.

Perpetuating factors are identified as either mechanical or systemic factors.

Mechanical perpetuating factors are ubiquitous, and systemic perpetuating factors are very common. Elimination of one or several, but not all, of the factors may provide only modest improvement in the therapeutic response until the remain-

*TP: trigger points

ing factors are resolved. The more thoroughly all significant perpetuating factors are managed, the more effective and longer lasting the treatment becomes.

Mechanical Perpetuating Factors. The columns in *Table 2* list specific mechanical perpetuating stresses juxtaposed beside the muscle or muscles most likely to be affected by each stress. Systemic perpetuating factors may relate to any or all skeletal muscles. Mechanical perpetuating factors include anatomical variations, seated and standing postural stress, life style and vocational stress.

Anatomic Variations: One common anatomic variation is a *short* leg and/or *small* hemipelvis,[134] which must be corrected by a heel lift and/or butt lift for lasting relief of low back[115] and sometimes head, neck and shoulder pain due to myofascial TPs.

The relatively common phenomenon of short upper arms is frequently an unrecognized perpetuator of TPs in the shoulder elevator muscles. This variation is corrected by providing elbow rests or pads that modify the furniture to fit the individual.[134]

The long 2nd metatarsal, or D.J. Morton foot configuration, throws the foot off balance due to the knife-edge effect during toe-off that disturbs gait and overloads lower extremity muscles. This is corrected by inserting a toe pad under the head of the 1st metatarsal bone.[134] [135]

Seated postural stress: This source of stress on the muscles may be induced by a hard smooth mat under an office chair, a chair seat too high for heels to reach the floor, the lack of a firm back support and persistent head-forward posture.

A *hard smooth mat*, such as plexiglass, makes the office chair with free castors glide readily whenever its occupant changes position or exerts the slightest pressure against the desk. The long toe flexors and intrinsic foot muscles try to grasp the slick floor; the effort overloads and perpetuates TPs in these muscles.

Another seated postural stress is caused by a chair seat too high for that individual's leg length, leaving the *heels dangling* off the floor. This causes under-thigh compression of the hamstrings and chronic shortening of the soleus muscle. Both effects are perpetuating factors for TPs and can be avoided by providing a suitable footrest (book, pillow or small footstool).

Sitting in a chair with the *back unsupported* may be caused by a seat that is too long from front to back, that is flat and provides no lumbar support, that supplies no scapular contact or that has a backrest with inadequate backward angulation. In a seat that is too long from front to back the calves encounter the front of the seat preventing the buttocks from reaching the backrest. The backrest should be contoured to support a normal lumbar lordosis. This also corrects the head-forward posture by correcting the thoracic kyphosis induced by an abnormally flattened back, thereby balancing the head erect over the shoulders without muscular effort. Scapular contact with the back-rest and backward angulation of the back-rest help to carry the weight of the head and shoulders and to stabilize the spine, relieving the quadratus lumborum and paraspinal muscles.

Standing postural stress: The *head-forward* posture is also induced by weight bearing on the heels and relieved, when standing, by shifting the center of gravity forward onto the balls of the feet, restoring the normal lumbar curve. This spinal posture permits the person to hold the head erect, balanced over the shoulders without muscle strain. It elevates the chest and restores normal postural relations by swinging the scapulae backward to their normal resting position and thus relieving the persistent shortening of the pectoral muscles.[134] This improved posture takes a major load off the posterior cervical muscles, which in the head-forward posture must hold the weight of head against the pull of gravity. To many neck and shoulder-girdle muscles, the head-forward posture is a powerful perpetuating factor that requires a major change in patient behavior.

A *canted running surface* is common on the slanted beach of the seashore or on a curved track. It produces the same effect as a short leg[134] that tilts the pelvis. The tilt must be compensated by the quadratus lumborum and/or paraspinal muscles, causing a persistent overload that perpetuates TPs in these muscles.

Vocational stress: Sustained *shoulder elevation* commonly overloads the upper trapezius and levator scapulae muscles, perpetuating their TPs. Typists and other workers using their hands in a relative fixed elevated position are prone to maintain their shoulders in a shrugged position to help elevate the hands to the level of their work. The work should be lowered or the patient's body raised.

Prolonged *arm abduction* similarly overloads the supraspinatus and deltoid muscles. Elbow support should be provided. Workers developed myofascial syndrome of the supraspinatus and upper trapezius muscles due to frequent repetitive movements stressing those muscles When tested, these painfully involved muscles had shorter duration of endurance and more rapid onset of electro-myographic evidence of fatigue than non-painful muscles.[44] The authors related their findings to alteration in muscle metabolism due to ischemia.

Overload of *hand supination* as when playing tennis or using a screw driver readily overloads the supinator muscle. The symptoms produced by active TPs in the supinator muscle are frequently labeled epicondylitis or tennis elbow. The arm should not be fully extended at the elbow when playing tennis, since that eliminates the forceful supinator function of the biceps brachii muscle.

Strong *grasp* overloads the finger extensors because vigorous extensor function is an essential part of grasp. Active TPs in these muscles tend to cause a painful and weak grip. Items are likely to slip out of the grasp unexpectedly due to unpredictable reflex inhibition. The supinator, the wrist and finger extensor muscles are commonly involved together.

Systemic Perpetuating Factors. Systemic perpetuating factors can aggravate TPs in any muscle and increase the irritability of all skeletal muscles rendering them more vulnerable to the development of secondary and satellite TPs.[134] Systemic factors include enzyme dysfunction, metabolic and endocrine dysfunction, chronic infection or infestation, and psychological stress.

Correction of a significant perpetuating factor reduces irritability of the muscles, which results in less pain and/or improved responsiveness of the muscles to specific myofascial therapy.

Muscle is an energy engine. It converts the energy of a high-energy molecule, adenosine triphosphate (ATP), to mechanical movement by converting it to a lower-energy molecule, adenosine disphosphate (ADP). Understandably, anything that interferes with energy metabolism of the muscle would tend to compromise this function and thereby would increase both muscle irritability and susceptibility to TPs.

Enzyme dysfunction: The nutritional inadequacies that most commonly perpetuate myofascial TPs are lack of B-complex vitamins, particularly B_1, B_6, B_{12} and folic acid. The detailed metabolic enzymatic functions and congenital deficiencies of each of these vitamins has been reviewed in detail.[134] Low electrolyte levels, potassium and calcium may be critical and minerals such as calcium, copper, and iron are essential. Vitamin *deficiency* is signaled by abnormally low laboratory values and by clinical symptoms that are ascribable to a lack of that vitamin. Vitamin

130

inadequacy is a suboptimal level, that may produce only a partial picture of deficiency or simply impair muscle function by increasing its irritability and tendency to develop TPs.

The prevalence of unrecognized vitamin *deficiency* is remarkably high, especially in hospital patients. Among 120 hospital patients, 88% had abnormally low levels in one or more of 11 vitamins.[4] Despite this high prevalence, the history of dietary intake was inadequate in only 39%. More than half of the patients were low in two or more vitamins. Serum folate, which was the commonest vitamin deficiency, was low in 45% of these patients. Symptoms of vitamin deficiency was clinically apparent in only 38% of these patients.[4] How many more of these patients had a vitamin *inadequacy* was not determined.

Clinical experience shows that the lower the serum value within the lower quartile of the "normal" range, the more likely it is that this degree of vitamin inadequacy contributes significantly to increased muscle irritability, and that it will require correction for lasting relief of that patient's chronic TP pain.

Vitamin dependence is observed in a few babies who are born with severe congenital deficiency of an enzyme that requires that vitamin as its coenzyme. Such defects require the ingestion of pharmacological megadoses of the vitamin to sustain life; the specific enzyme defects and their chemical recognition have been summarized for each of the B vitamins considered here.[134] However, unexplored is the prevalence of milder degrees of such congenital enzyme deficiencies that could multiply by many times the minimum vitamin requirement of individuals who have become progressively deficient in that enzyme as they reach middle age. The serum vitamin level might appear to be safely in the mid-normal range for these individuals. The wide range of individual variation in the requirements for essential nutrients including vitamins is well established.[140]

All of the B complex vitamins and vitamin C are water soluble. They have remarkably low toxicity because an excess is quickly excreted in the urine. This is not the case for the fat soluble vitamins A, D, and E, which readily accumulate to toxic levels. Vitamin A toxicity is not uncommon and can be a source of pain.

The common assumption that adequate dietary ingestion assures an adequate metabolic supply of a vitamin does not consider the many causes of vitamin insufficiency. They include not only inadequate ingestion of the vitamin, but also

131

impaired absorption, inadequate utilization, increased metabolic requirement and increased excretion or destruction within the body.[143] In addition, the usual selection process for individuals who serve as controls to establish normal values does not screen out individuals with marginal insufficiency, including many who show chemical evidence of vitamin deficiency and depletion of stores.[2] One should expect, therefore, that published normal values are not *optimal* values. This helps to explain why, clinically, the lower quartile of "normal" is often a zone of inadequacy for muscle metabolism.

A characteristic neurological finding in vitamin B_1 inadequacy is increasingly severe loss of vibration sense at progressively more distal sites on the upper and lower extremities. By comparing the time of loss of sensibility at successively more proximal levels following one activation of a long-period tuning fork, one can demonstrate progressively lower thresholds of response at successive proximal sites on the extremities.

The recommended daily allowance (RDA) for *Thiamine* (vitamin B_1) is dependent on the daily energy expenditure. The requirement for vitamin B_1 is greatest when carbohydrate is the source of energy. It is an essential enzyme for the entry of pyruvate (end-product of anaerobic metabolism) into the Krebs cycle for oxidative metabolism (the chief source of energy in muscle).[64] The critical symptoms of severe thiamine deficiency are recognized as wet beriberi (heart muscle failure) or dry beriberi that includes severe skeletal muscle weakness and serious central and peripheral nervous system dysfunction.[84]

Impressively so, *pyridoxine (vitamin B_6)* is a jack of all trades: an essential coenzyme to more than 60 enzymes in human metabolism. It is essential for the metabolism of numerous amino acids including the methionine to cysteine pathway, blockage of which leads to homocystinuria. It plays an important conformational or structural role in the enzyme phosphorylase. This enzyme is essential for the release of glucose from glycogen, which is a necessary first step for all anaerobic (glycolytic) metabolism in skeletal muscle. Pyridoxine is essential to the synthesis or metabolism of nearly all neurotransmitters. This correlates with the deterioration of mental function seen in experimental pyridoxine deficiency. It is required for the synthesis of nucleic acids, which are required for messenger RNA (ribonucleic acid) and, therefore, essential for normal cell reproduction. It is critical in the synthesis of at least 10 hormones including insulin and growth hormone.[134] This list is by no means complete.

Symptoms of vitamin B_6 deficiency include skin symptoms of dermatitis, glossitis and stomatitis; nervous system dysfunction that can lead to convulsions and peripheral neuritis; connective tissue swelling (carpal tunnel syndrome); and severe compromise of erythropoiesis that produces hypochromic anemia in experimental animals.[17] Several classes of drugs are well known to increase the demand for vitamin B_6. They include antitubercular drugs, oral contraceptives, the chelating agent penicillamine, anticonvulsants, corticosteroids, and excessive alcohol consumption.[134] Severe depletion of vitamin B_1 in chronic alcoholism is well recognized and is not uncommon in the heavy social drinker.

Both thiamine and pyridoxine are widely distributed in nature, but in limited amounts. Vitamin B_1 is rapidly destroyed by heat in neutral and alkaline solutions. It is stable in acidic solutions, but only to boiling temperature. Vitamin B_1 is quickly leached out of food during washing or boiling. Pyridoxine suffers substantial losses during cooking and is quickly destroyed by ultraviolet light (sunlight) and oxidation (when held on a steam table). Riboflavin (Vitamin B_2) and ascorbic acid (Vitamin C) are destroyed by fluorescent light.

Both *cobalamin (vitamin B_{12}) and folate* play an essential role in the synthesis of deoxyribonucleic acid (DNA) that is required for the maturation of erythrocytes and, therefore, for oxygen transport. Vitamin B_{12} is also essential for fat and carbohydrate metabolism; this may account for its importance to the integrity of the peripheral nervous system.[47]

Both vitamin B_{12} and folate deficiency characteristically cause megaloblastic anemia, but only vitamin B_{12} produces serious peripheral nervous system deficits. Many clinicians have been accustomed to basing vitamin therapy on the response of a patient's hematopoietic system. If the anemia is caused by vitamin B_{12} deficiency, but the patient is being treated with folic acid, the hematological picture will revert to normal with no improvement in, or even exacerbation of, the neurological deficits. This approach has lead to permanent neurological damage. For this reason, the Federal Drug Administration limits non-prescription folic acid to 400 micrograms per dose.

133

There is no need to guess. Laboratory testing for serum vitamin levels of both vitamin B_{12} and folate are readily available and usually leave no doubt as to what needs correction. Every chronic myofascial pain patient deserves these tests. Vitamin B_{12} tests err on the high side. The patient's serum level is likely to be lower, not higher, than the reported value.[134]

The metabolic interdependence of vitamin B_{12} and folate produces a reciprocal therapeutic effect. An example is the methyl folate trap in which folate metabolism is blocked for lack of vitamin B_{12}.[47] Folate may actually accumulate to unexpectedly high serum folate levels. Administration of vitamin B_{12} can precipitously drop the serum folate level and deplete what initially appeared to be an adequate reserve. A reverse effect may also be seen: a 20 or 30% drop in the serum vitamin B_{12} level following oral supplementation of badly needed folic acid.

Vitamin B_{12} is rarely deficient in the diet except in *strict* vegetarians. This vitamin is synthesized by bacteria and obtainable only in food products that have been contaminated by or have been affected by bacterial action. Source foods include practically all animal products and some legumes.[47]

An adequate serum cobalamin level is dependent on adequate ingestion, on gastric secretion of intrinsic factor, on adequate intestinal absorption (which is compromised by ileal disease), on reabsorption of much of the vitamin B_{12} that is secreted in the bile, and on adequate amounts of transport transcobalamines in the gut wall. Only if all of these are normal is daily ingestion of 3-5 micrograms of cobalamin sufficient.

Conversely, folates are widely distributed in many foods in modest amounts, particularly leafy green vegetables (foliage), and are very readily destroyed by processing and cooking. Folate is highly vulnerable to destruction by heat and oxidation; generally, 50-95% of the folate in food is destroyed in processing and preparation. Folate deficiency is the most common vitamin deficiency, especially in the elderly and those eating institutional cafeteria-style meals. Consistently over a period of years, three-fourths of the select group of patients referred to a chronic myofascial pain clinic had inadequate levels of vitamin B_{12} or folate (within the lower quartile of "normal" or lower).[110]

Serum levels of vitamins B_1 and B_6 are expensive and sometimes difficult to obtain. The vitamin B_{12} and folate tests are readily obtainable. Supplementation with 1-3 mg of folic acid daily, p.o., should bring the folate level to at least the mid-normal range within 2 or 3 weeks. A one mg (1000 ug) daily oral supplement of vitamin B_{12} will usually restore it to mid-range within 4 to 6 weeks, thus avoiding the necessity for injection. This dose is several hundred times the RDA, but totally innocuous. The administration of either vitamin B_{12} or folic acid alone can be hazardous because of their reciprocal relationship, unless the serum level of the other is safely above the mid-normal range. One cannot predict one vitamin inadequacy based on another, but the demonstrated inadequacy of one or several vitamins and temporary response to treatment should increase suspicion. The administration of a balanced B-complex supplement up to ten times RDA (B-50 dosage) should ensure that minor problems of diet, absorption and increased demand are met. Also, adverse interactions caused by excessive administration of one vitamin will be avoided. This philosophy of providing an excess is not applicable to the fat soluble vitamins A, D, and E. Quite the contrary, one source of increased muscular irritability appears to be above-normal serum vitamin A levels. Chronic MPS patients taking a *total* of more than 30,000 i.u. (including dietary intake) of vitamin A daily should have this serum level tested.

For different reasons, *absorbic acid (vitamin C)* is important to MPS patients. It is essential for hydroxalation of the amino acids lysine and proline to form the protocollagen molecule. Without it, the integrity of the connective tissue is compromised. In the absence of vitamin C to provide the collagen needed for strong vessel walls, the patient experiences marked capillary fragility and easy bruising. Capillary fragility leads to ecchymoses following injection of TPs. Ecchymoses are unsightly and irritating to the muscle.

Smoking markedly increases the oxidation of vitamin C, rapidly depleting it. One should beware of injecting TPs in smokers unless they have taken at least two grams of timed-release vitamin C daily for a minimum of 3 days prior to treatment.

Vitamin C is also of clinical importance to the muscles because 500 mg of timed-release vitamin taken at the time of excessive muscular activity can prevent much postexercise muscle soreness and stiffness.

Metabolic and endocrine dysfunction: The metabolic factors of gout, anemia, low electrolyte levels and hypoglycemia increase muscle irritability and symptoms from TPs, as do also the endocrine disturbances of hypometabolism and estrogen deficiency.

The monosodium urate crystals of *gout* are less soluble in the acidic media of injured tissues than in blood, and hence are deposited in areas of tissue injury and metabolic distress such as TPs. Patients with a gouty diathesis respond better to treatment when the hyperuricemia is under control, and generally respond better to injection than to stretch and spray. Vitamin C in relatively large amounts (one to four grams per day) is an innocuous and effective uricosuric agent.[57] The hyper-irritability of TPs in the muscles of some patients with serum uric acid levels in the high normal range subsides remarkably with uricosuric therapy.

From the muscle's point of view, *anemia* of any cause is a serious metabolic problem because the muscle depends on oxygen to sustain oxidative metabolism essential for meeting the bulk of its energy needs.

Abnormally *low electrolyte* levels of ionized calcium and potassium seriously disturb muscle function and increase muscle irritability, apparently because of their critical roles in the contractile mechanism. Serum ionized calcium is the essential measure. The total calcium that is ordinarily included in a blood chemistry profile correlates poorly with the ionized calcium.

The occurrence of *hypoglycemia* would intensify the metabolic distress of the muscle and it clearly aggravates myofascial TPs. Stretch or injection therapy should be deferred in patients while they are hypoglycemic, treatment then is likely to aggravate rather than relieve their symptoms. A packet of powdered soluble gelatin prepared as a drink is a handy source of available carbohydrate with enough protein to avoid a subsequent hypoglycemic reaction.

Evidence of *hypometabolism* is found in some treatment-refractory patients with persistent active myofascial TPs. Their serum folate levels should be up to at least the mid-normal range; this is important because folate inadequacy can cause symptoms resembling those of low thyroid function and is readily corrected. Confusion arises because laboratory tests of thyroid function are usually low normal and dismissed as being within normal limits. These patients have marginally low T3 uptake and low to midrange T_4 by radioimmune assay (RIA). In this group, insufficient thyroid function is revealed by a low basal metabolic rate[124] or a low basal body temperature,[6] by elevation of the serum cholesterol level and by the response to thyroid supplementation.

The basal temperature is obtained with an ovulation thermometer placed in the axilla daily by the patient for 10 minutes before arising after sleep. Normally, the basal temperature averages more than 36.1C (97.0F). The farther the basal temperature is below this value, the more vulnerable the patient is to hyperirritable TPs in the muscles and often to depression. Basal temperature in ovulating women is reached immediately after menses.

Sonkin[124] demonstrated that, with thyroid therapy, those patients needing supplemental thyroid consistently recovered their energy and positive outlook on life and had an increased basal metabolic rate with a decreased serum cholesterol value. Their muscles became less vulnerable to myofascial TPs and were more responsive to specific TP therapy. Travell corroborated these observations.[131]

Thyroid supplementation is contraindicated in patients with known cardiac arrhythmias or known myocardial disease that compromises cardiac reserve. Thyroid medication increases vitamin B_1 and estrogen requirements and may increase blood pressure. Overmedication causes symptoms of hyperthyroidism. Adjustment of dosage in these patients is dependent largely on clinical judgement and responses of basal metabolic rate and basal temperature. The site of metabolic dysfunction is apparently at the level of intracellular utilization and is poorly reflected in serum hormone levels.

Thyroid supplementation for those patients who meet the criteria described by Sonkin[124] remains controversial among endocrinologists, but of critical importance to those patients in whom this is a major perpetuating severe myofascial pain.

Chronic infection *and infestation:*Viral disease, bacterial infection and parasitic infestation can perpetuate MPS. During a systemic *viral illness*, including the common cold or attack of "flu," the irritability of myofascial TPs increases markedly. One of the most common sources is an outbreak of Herpes Simplex virus type I; however, neither Herpes Simplex virus type II (genital Herpes) nor Herpes Zoster are known to aggravate MPS. Herpes virus type I can cause the common aphthous mouth ulcer, canker sore, or cold sore. It may also appear on the skin of the body or extremities as isolated vesicles filled with clear fluid. Lesions have been reported in the esophagus, and the symptoms of vomiting and diarrhea strongly implicate gastrointestinal involvement comparable to that of the mouth.

No drug is known to cure Herpes Simplex Virus type I, but a multi-pronged attack can greatly reduce the frequency and severity of recurrences. A daily dose of 300-500 mg of niacinamide reinforces mucous membrane resistance. Three tablets (or 1 packet) of viable lactobacillis two or three times daily for at least a month helps to reestablish the normal intestinal bacteria, reducing the chance of an intestinal viral outbreak. Local therapy is applied by rubbing an antiviral ointment into the skin or mouth lesions 3 times daily, which accelerates resolution of the lesion.

Persistent *bacterial* infection tends to exacerbate muscle irritability. A chronic infection such as an abscessed tooth, infected sinus or chronic urinary tract infection can be a major perpetuating factor. Chronic sinusitis may arise from both infection and allergy. Normal erythrocyte sedimentation rate and C-reactive protein tests help to eliminate the possibility of chronic infection.

A *parasitic infestation* should be considered in travelers exposed to conditions of poor sanitation and among active homosexuals, as a likely perpetuator of myofascial pain. The worst offender is the fish tapeworm; next is giardiasis, and occasionally amebiasis. The first two tend to impair absorption of or consume vitamin B_{12} and the amoebae may produce myotoxins that are absorbed. The diagnosis of infestation is investigated by three stool examinations for occult blood, ova and parasites.

Post-traumatic hyperirritability syndrome: The group of myofascial pain patients with post-traumatic hyperirritability syndrome suffer greatly, are poorly understood and are difficult to help. They respond to strong sensory stimuli much differently than most patients. Following a major impact to the body and/or head, the muscles exhibit marked hyperirritability of TPs and a distressing vulnerability to strong sensory stimuli. The trauma has usually been an automobile accident or fall that was sufficiently severe to have inflicted some degree of damage to the sensory pathways of the central nervous system. These patients describe constant pain that is easily augmented by any strong sensory input including severe pain, a loud noise, vibration, prolonged physical activity and emotional stress. It may take days or weeks to recover from a degree of trauma or noise that to most people would be inconsequential. From the date of onset, coping with pain has suddenly

138

become the focus of life for these patients who previously paid no particular attention to pain. Their function is impaired by a marked increase in pain and fatigue if they exceed their restricted limit of activity.

One of the distinguishing characteristics of patients with the post-traumatic-hyperirritability syndrome is their loss of tolerance to what are to most people trivial mechanical stresses such as jarring, vibration, loud noises and mild bumps or thumps. Exposure to such a stimulus immediately produces an increase in the pain level. Most distinctive, the stimulus also causes a markedly increased sensitivity to subsequent stimuli so they suddenly become much more vulnerable to further aggravation of their misery. This increased arousal of the sensory system subsides slowly. It may take hours, days, or weeks—depending on the intensity of the stimulus—for this increased excitability of the sensory system to subside to its previous state. A strong sensory input appears to modulate the excitability of the arousal system. This increased excitability is paralleled by a corresponding increase in irritability of all of that patient's myofascial TPs.

The target area of TPs and pain tends to concentrate in the somatic distribution of the brainstem, cervical cord or lumbosacral cord. A few unfortunate individuals seem to have involvement of several regions. These patients are highly vulnerable to reinjury by additional trauma. It takes much less subsequent impact to exacerbate the whole process as compared to an initial accident.

The most effective treatment approach has been to inactivate all identifiable TPs and to correct perpetuating factors. On occasion, it may be necessary to reset the system by suppressing central nervous system excitability. To date, barbiturates have been found most effective.

Psychological stress: It is generally agreed that among chronic pain patients malingering is rare, a few percent at most.[51] Much controversy surrounds the question: "Is the chronic pain an expression of the patient's psychological dysfunctions or is the pain driving the patient crazy?" Patients who experience a serious chronic MPS that is undiagnosed and untreated are strongly impacted psychologically. They are confronted with a severe inescapable pain of unknown origin and of uncertain prognosis that is devastating their vocational, social and private lives. The future is an ominous, impenetrable dark cloud. The ensuing depression aggravates the pain and reinforces the uncertainty and sense of hopelessness.[51] The most valuable service to these patients is an unambiguous diagnosis of *treatable* MPS. They learn self-treatment and self-management techniques that give them control of the pain, rather than the pain controlling their lives and victimizing them.

As a positive prognostic factor for patients in chronic pain rehabilitation programs, the fact that they are still employed is much more important than the absence of litigation.[51] When patients reorient their primary focus of attention from being productive members of society to being pain patients, they develop a new self-image that shifts from function orientation to sickness orientation. It is of utmost importance to preserve the patient's vocational activity, if at all possible.

Reprinted with permission from Simons DG: Myofascial pain syndrome due to trigger points, chapter 45. Rehabilitation Medicine edited by Joseph Goodgold. C.V. Mosby Co., St. Louis, 1988 (pp. 686-723).

140

Appendix C

Yeast Questionnaire

Candida Questionnaire and Score Sheet

Section A of this questionnaire lists aspects of your medical history which may promote growth of the common yeast, *Candida Albicans*, and result in yeast-associated illness.

Section B and C evaluate the presence of symptoms which are often found in individuals who suffer from yeast-connected illnesses.

For each "yes" answer in Section A, circle the Point Score. Total the points and record the score in the box at the end of the section. Next, go to Sections B and C, and score as directed.

SECTION A: YOUR MEDICAL HISTORY

	Point Score
1. Have you been treated for acne with tetracycline, erythromycin, or any other antibiotics for one month or longer?	50
2. Have you ever taken antibiotics for any type of infection for more than two consecutive months, or in shorter courses four or more times in any 12-month period?	50
3. Have you ever taken an antibiotic—even for a single course?	6
4. Have you every had prostatitis, vaginitis, or other infections or problems with your reproductive organs for more than one month?	25
5. Have you been pregnant: Twice or more times?	5
Once?	3
6. Have you taken birth control pills for: More than two years?	15
Six months to two years?	8
7. Have you taken a corticosteroid such as prednisone, cortef, or medrol by mouth or inhaler for : More than two weeks?	15
Two weeks or less?	6
8. When you are exposed to perfumes, insecticides, or other chemicals, do you develop wheezing, burning eyes, or any other distress?	
Yes, and symptoms keep me from continuing my activities.	20
Yes, but symptoms are mild and do not change my activities.	5
9. Are your symptoms worse on damp or humid days, or in moldy places?	20
10. Have you ever had a fungal infection, such as jockitch, athlete's foot or of the nails or skin, which has been difficult to treat and lasted:	
More than two months	20
Less than two months	10
11. Do you crave any of the following: Sugar	10
Breads	10
Alcoholic Beverages	10
12. Does tobacco smoke cause you discomfort such as wheezing, burning eyes, or any other problem?	10

Total Score Section A _____

SECTION B: MAJOR SYMPTOMS

For each symptom which is present, enter the appropriate figure in the point score column. If a symptom is:

occasional or mild . . . . .3 points

frequent and/or moderately severe . . . . .6 points

severe and/or disabling . . . . .9 points

Add total score for this section and record it in the box at the end of this section.

Point Score

1. Fatigue or lethargy. _____

2. Feeling of being "drained." _____

3. Poor memory. _____

4. Feeling "spacey" or "unreal." _____

5. Inability to make decisions. _____

6. Numbness, burning, or tingling. _____

7. Insomnia. _____

8. Muscles aches. _____

9. Muscle weakness or paralysis. _____

10. Pain and/or swelling in joints. _____

11. Abdominal pain. _____

12. Constipation. _____

13. Diarrhea. _____

14. Bloating, belching or intestinal gas. _____

15. Troublesome vaginal burning, itching or discharge. _____

16. Prostatitis. _____

17. Impotence. _____

18. Loss of sexual desire or feeling. _____

19. Endometriosis or infertility. _____

20. Cramps and/or other menstrual irregularities. _____

21. Premenstrual tension. _____

22. Attacks of anxiety or crying. _____

23. Cold hands or feet and/or chilliness. _____

24. Shaking or irritable when hungry. _____

Total Score, Section B _____

SECTION C: OTHER SYMPTOMS*

For each symptom which is present, enter the appropriate figure in the point score column. If a symptom is:

occasional or mild . . . . .1 point

frequent and/or moderately severe . . . . .2 points

severe and/or persistent . . . . .3 points

Add total score for this section and record it in the box at the end of this section.

Point Score

1. Drowsiness.   _____
2. Irritability or jitteriness.   _____
3. Incoordination.   _____
4. Inability to concentrate.   _____
5. Frequent mood swings.   _____
6. Headache.   _____
7. Dizziness/loss of balance.   _____
8. Pressure above ears, feeling of head swelling.   _____
9. Tendency to bruise easily.   _____
10. Chronic rashes or itching.   _____
11. Psoriasis or recurrent hives.   _____
12. Indigestion or heartburn.   _____
13. Food sensitivity or intolerance.   _____
14. Mucus in stools.   _____
15. Rectal itching.   _____
16. Dry mouth or throat.   _____
17. Rash or blisters in mouth.   _____
18. Bad breath.   _____
19. Foot, hair or body odor not relieved by washing.   _____
20. Nasal congestion or post nasal drip.   _____
21. Nasal itching.   _____
22. Sore throat.   _____
23. Laryngitis, loss of voice.   _____
24. Cough or recurrent bronchitis.   _____
25. Pain or tightness in chest.   _____

26. Wheezing or shortness of breath. _____

27. Urinary frequency, urgency, or incontinence. _____

28. Burning on urination. _____

29. Spots in front of eyes or erratic vision. _____

30. Burning or tearing of eyes. _____

31. Recurrent infections or fluid in ears. _____

32. Ear pain or deafness. _____

While the symptoms in this section occur commonly in patients with yeast-connected illness, they also occur commonly in patients who do not have Candida.

Total Score Section A _____

Total Score Section B _____

Total Score Section C _____

Grand Total Score (add scores from Sections A, B and C) _____

The Grand Total Score will help you and your physician decide if your health problems are yeast-connected. Scores in women will run higher as 7 items in the questionnaire apply exclusively to them, while only 2 apply exclusively to men.

Yeast-connected health problems are almost certainly present in women with scores *over* 160, and in men with scores *over 140*.

Yeast-connected health problems are probably present in women with scores *over 120* and in men with scores *over 90*.

Yeast-connected health problems are possibly present in women with scores *over 60*, and in men with scores *over 40*.

With scores of *less than 60* in women and *40* in men, yeasts are less apt to cause health problems.

©1995, William Crook M.D., from his book Yeast Connection and The Woman, *Professional Books, Inc., Jackson, TN* (901) 423-5400. *Reprinted with permission.*

Appendix D

Information on Commonly Used Treatments for Chronic Fatigue Syndrome and Fibromyalgia

Nutritional Treatment

TwinLab Daily One Caps. This is an excellent multivitamin containing good levels of B-complex and other vitamins and minerals. Take one each morning. It will normally turn your urine bright yellow. If it upsets your stomach, take it with food, and/or at bedtime or switch to Centrum—one each morning instead. If the Centrum is well tolerated, try to add in a B complex vitamin, 50 mg, ½ tablet at a separate time of day. If problems still occur, let the doctor know. Taking a good multivitamin is critical.

Magnesium chloride or lactate. Magnesium is a mineral that is critical for helping tight muscles relax and for treatment of fatigue. The average American gets only 250-275 mg in their diet each day because of food processing. A normal diet (e.g. an Asian diet) supplies approximately 650 mg a day of magnesium. Magnesium is involved in over 80 different reactions in the body and is a critical supplement in treating CFS and Fibromyalgia. Since, magnesium oxide tablets are poorly absorbed, we often use magnesium chloride or lactate instead. It will take about eight months to replace magnesium deficits. After about eight months, you can decrease from six to two tablets a day.

Many people get diarrhea with magnesium. If this is a problem, take as much as your stomach will comfortably allow. Start with one or two tablets a day and work your way up.

Supermalic, Fibrocare and Ultramalic. These are a mixture of magnesium (see item 2 above) and malic acid. Malic acid is a food supplement that is found in citrus fruits. Studies have found that it helps energy metabolism in muscles and is helpful in Fibromyalgia.

L-carnitine. This is an amino acid (protein). It is available both over the counter and by prescription. As it is very expensive, we write it as a prescription so that people will have a better chance of getting it paid for by their insurance company. Several studies have shown that people with Chronic Fatigue Syndrome have very low muscle carnitine levels and that their fatigue often decreases and their energy improves after about six weeks of carnitine treatment. If your energy improves, continue at the lowest dose it takes to maintain the improvement. If there is no change after six weeks, stop the carnitine.

Coenzyme Q10. This is another food supplement that is used by the muscles for energy. It is available through health food stores. It is also somewhat expensive, and therefore we recommend that you send away for it wholesale. The CFIDS Buyers Club occasionally has the 200 mg oil-based sublingual tablet on sale. Some experts feel the oil-based tablets are absorbed better.

Iron. "Normal" levels for iron are adequate to prevent anemia but not adequate to prevent other signs of iron deficiency (including fatigue). We recommend several brands of iron. Ferrous-Sequels has a stool softener which decreases the tendency for constipation. Most people also find Chromagen is well tolerated. Chromagen also has the benefit of being a prescription drug and therefore sometimes is covered by insurance. Vitron C has a lower dose but is easier on the stomach. Iron will cause constipation and will often turn your stools black. This is normal. It is important not to take any iron supplements (except for the 10 mg in the TwinLab multivitamin) within six hours of sleep medications or thyroid (and, perhaps, other hormonal supplements), or you will not absorb the medication.

B-12. This is a very important vitamin in chronic fatigue and Fibromyalgia. Although current normal levels are adequate to prevent anemia, numerous studies show that deficiencies can cause severe neurologic and psychologic dysfunction at levels that are well within what is traditionally considered the normal range. Because of this, we recommend treatment with B-12 shots any time the B-

12 level is less than 540 pg/ml. Although oral B-12 supplements in high dose (e.g. 1000 mcg a day) will slowly raise the B-12 levels, this can take years. Because of this, we recommend a series of B-12 shots to initially raise levels. After this, most patients find that the multivitamin is adequate to maintain their B-12 levels.

Hormonal Supplements

Synthroid. This is the main form that thyroid hormone takes in the body (T4). Many people have an underactive thyroid despite technically normal blood tests and often get dramatic relief from treating these subclinical thyroid deficiencies. The dosing that we use is usually very low and will usually not cause any side effects. Rarely, one can see caffeine-like side effects (e.g. shakiness or palpitations) if the dose is a little too high. If this occurs, I would cut back the dose. If somebody has underlying angina, the thyroid can unmask this. Because of this, I would stop the Synthroid and call your doctor immediately if any chest pain occurs. This is very rare, we have never seen it with the low dosing that we are using. Take thyroid hormones in the morning.

Armour Thyroid. This is the natural thyroid, and it contains a mixture of the two most common thyroid hormones (T3 and T4) in the body. Both this and the synthetic thyroid (see item 1 above) are best taken in the morning. Side effects are the same as Synthroid. Still people who don't improve with one form of thyroid can often still dramatically improve with the other.

Cortef. This is an adrenal hormone (cortisol). When low, people will often feel fatigued, unable to deal with stress, and get recurrent infections that take a long time to resolve. Low cortisol is also associated with hypoglycemic symptoms and lightheadedness. The dosing that we are using is a very low dose and usually not associated with side effects, except for the occasional acid stomach. In higher dosing, one can see an unmasking of a tendency to high blood pressure and diabetes as well as seeing osteoporosis and other severe side effects. These are rarely seen in doses under 35 mg a day. During periods of physical stress (e.g. colds), it would be prudent to double the cortef dose for four to five days. We should certainly be notified if you are sick, undergoing any surgery, or other major problems.

DHEA. This is another adrenal hormone that is often low in Chronic Fatigue Syndrome. It is the hormone that the adrenal makes the most of. We are also just learning about its function in the human body. DHEA normally decreases with age. Low DHEA levels are associated with increased risk of heart disease, diabetes, and possibly cancer. Higher levels are associated with longer life and a sense of well being. Research has shown that if levels are low, people will often feel fatigued. Patients often feel much better with treatment. Side effects on this hormone are also rare. Occasionally, there is some acne or an increase in hair growth on the extremities and, rarely, even on the face. It is important that we monitor the blood levels to make sure that they are in the optimum range. With this hormone and with Cortef, people will usually know if it is going to be helpful within two to three weeks. It can only be obtained by telephone from a few pharmacies.

Florinef. This is a hormone that helps to conserve salt and water. Many patients find that they have increased thirst and a tendency to low blood pressure and dizziness. Recent research shows that many of the symptoms of Chronic Fatigue Syndrome can improve with Florinef treatment. It can take up to three months to see the full benefit. Start slowly with ¼ of a .1 mg tablet each morning. Increase to ½ tablet daily the second week, ¾ tablet daily the third week, and then one each morning. Get plenty of salt, water, and extra potassium (e.g. bananas, V-8 juice).

149

Oxytocin. This is a hypothalamic/pituitary hormone and neurotransmitter. It is most often thought of as the hormone that induces labor. Although we are just learning what its role is in other body functions, some researchers have found that patients feel better with Oxytocin treatment. If this is the case, improvement will usually occur within two weeks. The dose that we use is a dose that has been reported to be normally put out by the body during orgasm. There is no blood test to test for Oxytocin levels, and, therefore, treatment is given if symptoms exist suggestive of Oxytocin deficiency. These symptoms are cold hands, cold feet, pallor (being pale), decreased short-term memory, as well as many other common symptoms seen in CFS and Fibromyalgia.

Choline and inositol. Taking 1500 mg/day of each daily (beginning six weeks before the Oxytocin) can make the Oxytocin more effective. Side effects with these are rare.

Anti-Fungal Treatments

Nystatin. This is a very benign antifungal. The medication itself rarely causes side effects (except perhaps mild nausea), because it is not absorbed into the body in the doses we use (i.e. it stays in the bowel and is excreted). When people have yeast overgrowth and the yeast is rapidly killed off, you can see a flaring of the symptoms. Because of this, we recommend that you start the treatments slowly and increase the daily dose by one tablet every one to four days until you are up to the recommended dosing. If the symptoms do flare, cut back on the dosing until you are comfortable and then slowly increase the dosing again. We usually recommend that people stay on Nystatin for about five months to help to clear any yeast overgrowth in the bowel. Unfortunately, the concept of yeast overgrowth is a very controversial one, and there are no definitive tests to define the difference between normal yeast growth and overgrowth. This would be similar to not being able to distinguish between the normal amount of yeast that we see in our skin versus a condition like athlete's foot or thrush. We can see skin conditions. When the overgrowth is inside the body, we wind up having to treat based on suspicion of a problem. The stool test and the questionnaire that you filled out will help us to determine whether you are at high-risk for a yeast overgrowth.

Sporanox (itraconazole) and Diflucan. These are very powerful yet safe anti-fungals. Unfortunately, they are also very expensive. Most of the studies done in the United States using these treatments were done on terminal AIDS patients. These patients get horrible side effects from almost anything (e.g. they can die from taking a common sulfa antibiotic). In European studies on patients with moderate yeast overgrowth without AIDS, the side effect profile showed it to be a very safe agent. Once in a rare while, liver inflammation can occur. We have not seen this, however, with Sporanox. It is important to take the Sporanox or Diflucan with food or else you will loose about 40 percent of the absorption. If you are taking two tablets a day, they should be taken together. We usually recommend that people take it for six weeks (while on the Nystatin) and then stop. If the symptoms improve quite a bit on the Diflucan or Sporanox, and then recur when they are stopped, we usually will repeat a six-week course.

Milk Bacteria. e.g. acidophilus or lactobacillus. Take 3-6 billion units daily.

These compete with the yeast.

Antiparasitics

Flagyl. This is a common antiparasitic agent. Its main side effect is nausea. This is not dangerous, but it can be a nuisance. Do not drink alcohol while you are taking Flagyl or you will vomit. You may feel worse for one to three weeks while the parasites die off.

Yodoxin. This is an antiamebic. The main side effect we usually see is mild nausea.

Artemesia and Tricyclin. These are antiparasitic herbal remedies. The main, but uncommon, side effect is nausea. Artemesia is taken 500 mg two capsules three times a day for 20 days. Tricyclin is taken two tablets three times a day after meals for six to eight weeks.

Sleeping Aids

DO NOT DRIVE WHILE YOU ARE SEDATED FROM ANY MEDICINE

Begin with a low dose (e.g. ⅛-1 tablet) and work your way up to a dose that causes you to sleep through the night without being too sedated the next day. Initially take it earlier (e.g. 7 p.m.) so the sedation wears off earlier the next day. The next day sedation usually goes away in two to three weeks. If you can not take the medication, call the doctor so you can try another one.

Elavil (amitriptyline). At doses up to 300 mg/day, Elavil is used as an antidepressant and for nerve injury. We use it for Fibromyalgia because it increases the deeper states of sleep that patients are lacking. We also use a very tiny dose compared to the dose used for other illnesses. The medication is not addictive. It is often very sedating however. Sedation can be decreased by starting with a very low dose (5-10 mg) and slowly working your way up until you are getting a good solid night's sleep without being too hung-over the next day. The main side effects include dry mouth, constipation, mild weight gain, and, rarely, difficulty with urinating. Do not use more than 100 mg/night without checking with your doctor.

Flexeril (cyclobenzaprine). This is a muscle relaxant. The usual dose is one tablet three times a day. We use it here predominantly to help normalize the sleep cycle. The dose for sleep is one-half to two tablets at bedtime. The main side effects are sedation and dry mouth. Mild weight gain can be seen with Flexeril or Elavil.

Desyrel (trazodone). This is usually used (at doses of 300 mg a day) as a calming agent. It is not addictive and it is sedating. Rarely, males can have prolonged erections (over an hour) that will not subside. If this occurs your doctor should be called immediately.

Herbal remedies. These can be very helpful and nonaddictive. They include valerian, passiflora, lemon balm (*Melissa officinalis*), hops, and camomile among others. These are generally considered to be very safe agents.

Melatonin. This is a naturally occurring hormone that helps regulate the day/night cycle. It is available in health food stores. It should only be taken in the evening. The usual dose is 3-6 mg/night. Some studies have found a dose as low as .3 mg to be effective.

Soma. This muscle relaxant is usually taken three to four times a day to treat muscle spasm. It can also be used one tablet at night time to help sleep.

Klonopin. This is a very powerful muscle relaxant. It is mildly addictive and, therefore, we save it for our more severe cases. It is very sedating and needs to be started at a very low dose (e.g. ¼-1 tablet at bedtime). The medication can be increased by ¼-½ mg every three days to a total of 2 mg a day (it is sometimes used in doses much higher than this, but this should not be done without first consulting with your doctor). If muscle spasm is severe, it can be taken three to four times during the day. If sleep is a major problem, then it should be taken predominantly at bedtime.

Ambien. This is a sleeping pill. The usual dose is 5-20 mg at bedtime. It does not worsen the sleep cycle like other sleeping pills and does not appear to be addictive (even though the FDA requires that they list this as a side effect). It causes less side effects then most of the other sleep medications listed above.

152

Other Agents

Zoloft, Prozac, Paxil, Serzone and Effexor. These are nonaddictive antidepressant agents. These agents tend to increase the body's serotonin levels (a neurotransmitter). They are usually not sedating, but often have an energizing effect, even in the absence of depression. Because of this, they can be useful in the absence of depression in helping fatigue. They also should be taken in the morning as they can keep people awake if they are taken in the evening. Some people might be sedated by the medication, in which case it is appropriate that they take it at night. Some people experience delayed orgasm on these. This is less likely with serzone.

If you get too shaky when you take the medication, start slowly (e.g. ½-¼ tablet) and slowly increase it by ¼-½ tablet every week. The maximum dose on these medications is usually two to four tablets daily. Do not increase the dose beyond what the doctor has recommended without first getting the doctor's approval. It takes six weeks to see the medication's full effect.

Nitroglycerin, nimodipine, mexiletine, hydralazine, Zantac, etc... are often used for other medical problems, but have been found to sometimes be helpful in Fibromyalgia and Chronic Fatigue Syndrome. As these are used less frequently, the doctor will discuss these agents with you if and when they are prescribed.

Appendix D (Part 2)

Treatment Protocol—CFS/Fibromyalgia

Dear Patient,

Below is a listing of some of the more common treatments used in treating Chronic Fatigue Syndrome and Fibromyalgia. See the information sheet for more information about these specific treatments.

NUTRITIONAL TREATMENTS

_____ 1. TwinLab Daily One Caps (with)(without) iron, one each morning. Take with food if your stomach is upset.

_____ 2. Magnesium chloride, two tablets three times a day for eight months, and then two a day (less if diarrhea is a problem). Start with one a day and slowly increase the dose.

_____ 3. Supermalic, Fibrocare or Ultramalic, two to three tablets two or three times a day for eight months, then two to four tablets a day (less if diarrhea is a problem).

_____ 4. L-carnitine, 1000 mg three times a day.

_____ 5. Coenzyme Q10, _____ mg _____ times a day.

_____ 6. Calcium, 500-1000 mg daily (a chewable calcium or Os-Cal or Caltrate is recommended).

_____ 7. Ferrous Sequels (iron), one tablet _____ times a day. Do not take within six hours of any hormone tablets.

_____8. Chromagen, (iron) one tablet _____ times a day. Do not take within six hours of any hormone preparations, as this can prevent their absorption.

_____9. Vitamin B-12, one shot (1000 mcg) weekly for _____ weeks.

SLEEPING AIDS FOR FIBROMYALGIA

_____ 1. Elavil (amitriptyline), 10 mg, one-half to five at bedtime.

_____ 2. Flexeril (cyclobenzaprine), 10 mg, ½-2 at bedtime.

_____ 3. Desyrel (trazodone), 50 mg, ½-6 at bedtime.

_____ 4. Ambien, 10 mg, ½-2 at bedtime.

_____ 5. Super Snooze (herbal sleep remedy), 1-3 at bedtime.

_____ 6. Valerian root (herbal sleep remedy), 360-450 mg—one at bedtime.

_____ 7. Melissa (lemon balm), 80-160 mg plus Valerian 180-360 mg (available from To Your Health. Called Valerian Rest. *See Appendix K.*)

_____ 8. Melatonin (available at health food stores), 3 mg, one to two at bedtime.

_____ 9. Klonopin, ½mg, begin slowly and work your way up as sedation allows. One-half tablet at bedtime increasing up to four tablets at bedtime.

_____ 10. Soma, ½-1 at bedtime.

HORMONAL TREATMENTS

_____1. Synthroid, _____ mcg one each morning (do not take within six hours of an iron supplement except for the iron in your multivitamin).

_____2. Armour Thyroid, _____ grain _____ tablets each morning.

_____3. Cortef, 5 mg tablets _____ tablet(s) at breakfast, _____ at lunch, _____ tablet(s) at 4 p.m.

_____4. DHEA _____ mg each morning.

_____5. Florinef, 0.1 mg, one each morning. Begin with ¼ tablet and increase by ¼ tablet each three to seven days. Increase more slowly if headache occurs.

_____6. Oxytocin, 10 units each morning

_____7. Choline and inositol, 500 mg of each three times a day (available at health food stores).

ANTI-YEAST TREATMENTS

_____1. Avoid sweets, this includes sucrose, glucose, fructose, corn syrup, or any other sweets until the doctor says that it is okay to include them in your diet again. Avoid fruit _juices_, which are naturally sweet. Having one to two fruits a day (the whole fruit as opposed to the juice) is okay.

_____2. Acidophilus or other milk bacteria, three to six billion units/day (refrigerated). Take with milk if able.

_____3. Nystatin, 500,000 units, two tablets four times a day. Begin with one a day and increase by one tablet a day until you are up to the total dose. Your symptoms may initially flare as the yeast die off. If this occurs increase the Nystatin slowly or stop for awhile until symptoms decrease. The Nystatin is usually taken for five months.

_____4. Diflucan or Sporanox, 100 mg, begin this four weeks after beginning the nystatin. Take two each day (simultaneously) with food for six weeks. If the symptoms have improved and then worsen when you stop the Sporanox, refill the prescription for another six weeks. (Note: A six-week supply costs over $500!) If your symptoms flared when you began the Nystatin, begin with one-half to one capsule a day for the first week.

TREATMENT FOR STOOL PARASITES

_____1. Flagyl (metronidazole), _____ mg three times a day for _____ days. Do not drink alcohol while on this medication as it will make you vomit.

_____2. Yodoxin, 650 mg three times a day for 20 days.

_____3. Artemesia annua (an herbal antiparasitic), 500 mg, two tablets three times a day for 20 days.

_____4. Tricyclin (an herbal antiparasitic), two capsules three times a day after meals for six to eight weeks.

NONSPECIFIC TREATMENTS

_____ 1. Nitroglycerin, ¼-1 tablet dissolved under the tongue as needed for muscle pain.

_____ 2. Rhus tox (homeopathic treatment), dissolve under the tongue as directed on the bottle.

_____ 3. Naphazoline hydrochloride, 0.1%, one drop in each eye, four times a day as needed.

_____ 4. Nimodipine, 30 mg _____ times a day.

_____ 5. Mexiletine, 150 mg _____ times a day.

_____ 6. Pyridostigmine, 30 mg _____ times a day.

_____ 7. Hydralazine (Apresoline), 10-25 mg _____ times a day.

_____ 8. Zantac, 150 mg twice a day.

_____ 9. Zoloft, _____ mg, _____ tablet(s) each morning.

_____ 10. Paxil, 20 mg, _____ tablet(s) each morning.

_____ 11. Prozac, 20 mg, _____ tablet(s) each morning.

_____ 12. Effexor, 37½ mg _____ times a day.

_____ 13. Serzone, 100 mg 2 times a day for 1 week, then 150 mg 2 times a day.

157

Appendix E
Adrenal Gland Test

Welcome to Your Cortrosyn Stimulation Test

The cortrosyn stimulation test is a test to check the ability of your adrenal gland to respond to the everyday stresses of life. The adrenal gland helps us respond to infections, physical stresses, psychological stresses, and the other traumas that we encounter in our day-to-day lives. Increasingly, evidence is mounting that many people are chronically fatigued because their adrenal gland is underactive. This can occur by the destruction of the gland or because of the excessive stress put on the gland by the chronic infections often seen in Chronic Fatigue Syndrome. If this is the case, supplying adrenal hormone can cause a significant improvement in the way people feel, as well as increase their ability to fight infections and deal with other stresses.

The test itself takes about an hour and a half. The nurse will initially draw your blood to check the level of a hormone (cortisol) that your adrenal gland makes. This will be followed by an injection of a hormone that the body normally produces to stimulate the adrenal gland. The hormone is very similar to what your body makes every day and is less than a body would normally make for many day-to-day stresses. Generally there are no side effects from this shot, although occasionally people with an underactive adrenal gland will find that they feel better or worse for a few days. The nurse will draw your blood in a half-hour and again in another half-hour to see how your adrenal gland responds to the hormone's message to make more adrenal hormone (cortisol). If your body is unable to increase cortisol production adequately in response to the hormone shot, the adrenal is not working properly and treatment is then recommended. In some cases people have a borderline response. Then we recommend a trial treatment for six weeks to see if it improves functioning and energy. We are finding it is very common for people with an underactive adrenal to have vitamin B-12 deficiency and an underactive thyroid gland. This is not surprising since a damaged immune system (autoimmunity) is a common cause of these three conditions. Please let me know if you have any questions.

Preparation for the Test:
- No caffeine for 24 hours prior to the test. This includes coffee, tea, colas, etc., and all "decaffeinated" beverages.
- It is best not to have breakfast on the day of the test; but if needed, you may have toast and juice.

Best wishes,
Jacob E. Teitelbaum, M.D.

Appendix E (Part 2)
How to Use Cortef

Instructions

The medication you have been prescribed is a normal adrenal hormone. In the dosage that you will be taking, it will usually not cause an excess of hormone in your body or the side effects that result from such an excess. The tablets taste somewhat bitter. If they are taken on an empty stomach, they may cause gastric discomfort and indigestion. It may be helpful, therefore, to take them with milk or an antacid. If you have had a peptic ulcer (of the stomach or duodenum), take food or an antacid with each dose. If the medication keeps you up at night, take the entire dose by noon.

Take _____ 5 mg cortef tablet(s) with breakfast, _____ at noon, _____ at 4 p.m. and _____ at bedtime, for a total of _____ tablets daily. It may be taken before, during, or after meals, but most patients prefer to take it just before meals. If meals are delayed or missed, try to take the medication at the usual mealtime. If you forget to take a dose, for example, at lunchtime, and think of it in the middle of the afternoon, take it when you think of it. If you do not remember it until the next dose is due, take both doses at the same time in order to have the correct total dosage for the day. It will not be harmful to double up on doses, but the medication will be more effective if you take each dose at its proper time. It is helpful to have a small pill box in which you put each day's dosage each morning. Carry it with you. This not only reminds you to take the medication, but also will enable you to determine whether you have taken a dose. Do not stop the medication suddenly. When the hormone is tapered off, decrease the last dose each day. First decrease by one-half to one tablet each one to four weeks until the optimum dose is reached, or you are off the cortef. The morning dose is the last one to be stopped.

Because this is a normal hormone, it will not interfere with your other medication. If you should develop any major stress, such as surgery, or a cold or influenza, double each dose and telephone your doctor. You should also take any other medication prescribed by us and may take aspirin, antihistamines, decongestants, antibiotics, or cough medicine. The increased dose of this medication should be continued until you have recovered from the stress or infection. Then return to your previous dosage. Call the doctor if this takes more than two weeks.

If any other questions arise, be sure to call your doctor's office.

Jacob E. Teitelbaum, M.D.

Appendix F

Treating Respiratory Infections Without Antibiotics
Jacob Teitelbaum, M.D.

Winter Colds and Flu

The cold and flu season is rapidly approaching, and prevention is important.

WHAT CAN I DO TO PREVENT COLDS?

When flu and other epidemics roll through town, most people will come in contact with the viruses. By keeping up your defenses you can often avoid catching the infection. This means eating right and getting enough rest. For people over 65, as well as those of any age with heart, lung, and other significant illnesses or people who have a lot of contact with the public, taking the flu vaccine can be helpful.

Less than 5 percent of the population gets the RDA of all of the vitamins and minerals they need. This results in decreased resistance to infections. Vitamins A, C, E, folate, and zinc are especially important here. I recommend most people (without significant problems) take a Twin Lab Daily One capsule vitamin (without iron). When infections are prevalent in a community, adding 500 to 1000 mg a day of vitamin C will also boost your immunity.

WHAT IF I CATCH A RESPIRATORY INFECTION?

Respiratory infections come in many types. Those in the nose and sinuses are often called sinusitis. Those in the chest are called bronchitis or, if more extensive, they can become pneumonia If your mucus is yellow or green through the day, this suggests a bacterial infection. In this case antibiotics (combined with the treatment below) can help speed healing. If the mucus is clear or white, this most often reflects a viral infection and will not likely benefit from antibiotics. There are two common important exceptions to this: One is sore throat, in which case strep throat should be considered; the other is severe lung congestion, in which case "walking pneumonia" (which responds to erythromycin antibiotics) or viral pneumonia should be considered.

The following will help your respiratory infections resolve more quickly:

1. Zinc lozenges, (must have *at least* 10-20 mg of zinc per lozenge)—suck on one lozenge five to eight times a day until the cold improves. This speeds up the healing of colds by about 40 percent.

2. Vitamin C—take one gram (1,000 mg) four to eight times a day (less if diarrhea and gas become a problem).

3. Drink *plenty* of water and hot, caffeine-free teas.

4. If you have a flu-like illness (fever, chills, achiness, malaise, etc.) taking a homeopathic remedy called Oscillococcinum speeds healing and will help you be more comfortable. This is most effective if started early in the infection.

5. If the infection is in the nose, using nasal rinses can be very helpful (they only sound gross!). To do this, dissolve ½ teaspoon of salt in a cup of lukewarm water. Inhale some of the solution through your nose. This can be done using a baby nose bulb or an eye dropper (while laying down), or sniffing it out of the palm of your hand while standing by a sink. Then *gently* (so you don't hurt your ears) blow your nose and repeat with the other nostril. You are only sniffing the water about one inch up into your nostrils (no need to choke yourself!). Repeat this until the nose is clear. This washes out 90 percent of the infection and makes it much easier for your body to heal. Do this at least twice a day and gargle with the salt water that is left in the cup.

6. Take Tylenol for muscle aches and use Cepacol or Chloraseptic for sore throats. The above salt water gargle also helps the sore throat.

7. If you are on antibiotics, avoid sweets and take refrigerated lactobacillus capsules (milk bacteria) or eat one cup of yogurt with live culture daily (e.g. Dannon) to lessen the severity of yeast overgrowth.

8. The herbal immune stimulant Echinacea can enhance your body's defenses. Use

163

50 drops (~1 dropperful) or 300-400 mg of the dry extract three times a day. Goldenseal is also helpful.

The above supplements are available at most health food stores. May the cold bugs pass you by!

Best wishes on your continued health.

Appendix G

Stool Test Specimen Collection*

Before taking the Fleet's Phospho Soda, collect a stool specimen and place 1 tsp. into the bottle with the white cap and pink liquid. Then take the laxative to obtain a purged specimen.

FOR PURGE (READ INSTRUCTIONS CAREFULLY BEFORE STARTING)

The purpose of the stool purge is to get the best possible stool sample to check for bowel parasites and yeast. The routine random tests being done in almost all standard labs are generally not adequate or reliable.

The objective of the stool purge is to secure a watery, loose sample. This pulls the organisms off the intestinal walls so they may be detected.

For a.m. Purge. Eat a very light meal the evening before. No breakfast the morning of the purge.

For p.m. or Evening Purge. No dinner until all specimens are done. You may eat a regular dinner afterwards.

To begin the purge, you will need to drink the entire (1½ oz.) bottle of Fleets Phospho Soda. The laxative is very salty tasting and you may wish to dilute it with water or juice. Do not collect the first few specimens if they are not "watery" or loose. Normally this may take about two hours.

*These are the directions we use in our office for our stool specimen test. Your doctor may use another procedure.

Remember to look for any blood, mucus, or anything unusual when collecting the specimen.

A helpful hint in collecting the specimen is to make a bowl of tin foil and place it on top of the water in the toilet. You can then use the little scoop inside the vial or use a plastic spool to collect enough of the specimen to raise the level of the liquid in the vial to the red line. Do not collect a specimen that has contacted the toilet water.

Both specimens should be returned to the lab as soon as possible. (Within a few days.)

166

Appendix H
Nasal Congestion Rx

Dr. Alexander Chester recommends trying the following therapeutic trial for nasal congestion/sinusitis:

1. Keflex (500 mg four times a day) for one week followed by doxycycline (100 mg two times a day) for one week if there is no improvement (prescription antibiotics).
2. Xylometazoline .1% nasal spray, three times a day, for three days (prescription).
3. Sudafed 60 mg, four times a day, or 120 mg (sustained release), two times a day (may cause shakiness or palpitations).
4. Nasal steam inhalations, 20 minutes, three times a day.
5. Sleep eight hours a night.
6. No beer, wine, or milk products.

Appendix I
Patient Support Groups

I strongly recommend you join the national support group. It is the *best* patient support group I've seen for any illness.

CFIDS Association of America

P.O. Box 220398

Charlotte, NC 28222-0398

(800) 442-3437

A membership form is included at the end of Appendix I.

There are also many excellent regional groups:

American Association for CFS	P.O. Box 895, Olney, MD 20830 *An umbrella organization focusing on scientific research*
Arthritis Foundation	P.O. Box 19000, Atlanta, GA 30326 (800) 283-7800
Candida Research Foundation	1638 B Street, Hayward, CA 94541 (510) 582-2179
CFIDS Activation Network (CAN)	P.O. Box 345, Larchmont, NY 10538 (212) 627-5631

| **CFIDS Pathfinder** | P.O. Box 2644, Kensington, MD 20891-2644 |
| | (301) 530-8624 |

CFIDS Association of America P.O. Box 220398, Charlotte, NC 28222-0398
(800) 442-3437

CFIDS Society, Linda Coffey, Group Leader
South Coast Chapter 5200 Heil Ave, #23
Huntington Beach, CA 92647

CFS Association of Virginia, Inc. P.O. Box 2337, Glen Allen, VA 23058-2337
(804) 330-7518

CFS Crisis Center 27 W 20th St., Ste 703, New York, NY 10011
(212) 691-4800 Fax (212) 691-5113

CFS Foundation 10 Wild Partridge Court
Greensboro, NC 27455
(919) 288-2893, (800) 597-4237

CFS Hotline (800) Help-CFS

CFS/ME Computer P.O. Box 11347, Washington, DC 20008

Networking Project Internet e-mail: cfs-me@sjuvm,stjohns.edu

Chicago CFS Association 818 Wenonah Ave, Oak Park, IL 60304
(708) 524-9322

Chronicles of CFIDS John Friedrich, P.O. Box 465
Ashland, MA 01721

Compuserve CFIDS CFS/CFIDS/FMS Section (16)
Support Area Health & Fitness Forum (Good Health)
CFIDS Info: (505) 898-4635
Compuserve Info: (800) 898-8199

Connecticut CFIDS Association P.O. Box 9582, Forestville, CT 06011
(203) 582-3437 (582-CFIDS)

169

Environmental Health Association/HEAL	Chapter, 1800 S. Robertson Blvd., Suite 380 Los Angeles, CA 90035 (213) 837-2048
Essex County FM Group	977 University Ave., W 2nd Fl. Windsor, Ont., Canada N9A 5S3 (519) 254-0417
Fibromyalgia Association British Columbia	Box 15455, Vancouver, B.C. Canada V6B 5B2 (604) 540-0488
Fibromyalgia Association of Greater Washington	P.O. Box 2373 Centreville, VA 22020 (703) 790-2324
Fibromyalgia Association of Northern VA	(703) 912-1727
Fibromyalgia Association of Texas, Inc.	5650 Forest Lane, Dallas, TX 75230 (214) 363-2473
Fibromyalgia Network	5700 Stockdale Hwy, #100 Bakersfield, CA 93309 (805) 631-1950
FM Association of Central Ohio	Riverside Hospital, Ste 8, 3545 Olentangy River Rd., Columbus, OH 43214 (614) 262-2000
FM Association of Florida, Inc.	P.O. Box 14848, Gainesville, FL 32604-4848 (904) 373-6865
Food Allergy Network	747 Holly Ave., Fairfax, VA 22030-5647 (800) 929-4040
Greater New York CFS Coalition	880 Pine Ave, West Islip, NY 11795 (516) 548-8237

Gulf Coast CFS/CFIDS Association	752 J Avenue Estancias Venice, FL 34292-2316 (813) 484-0706
Los Angeles CFIDS Association	P.O. Box 5414, Sherman Oaks, CA 91413 (818) 785-8301 (818) 458-9092 *(recorded info line)*
Massachusetts CFIDS Association	808 Main Street, Waltham, MA 02154 (617) 893-4415
M.E. Association of Canada	246 Queen St., Suite 400 Ottawa, Ontario, K1P 5E4 Canada (613) 563-1565
National CFS Hotline	Charleston, SC (800) 237-2407
National CFS and Fibromyalgia Association (NCFSFA)	3521 Broadway, Suite 222 Kansas City, MO 64111 (816) 931-4777
National Organization for SAD (Seasonal Affective Disorder)	P.O. Box 40133, Washington, DC 20016
Nightingale Research Foundation	383 Danforth Ave. Ottawa, Ontario K2A OE3 Canada
Ontario Fibrositis Association	250 Bloor St. E, #401 Toronto, Canada M4W 3P2 (416) 967-1414
Rhode Island CFIDS Association	UPC Building 500 Prospect St Pawtucket, RI 02860 (401) 729-0019

San Francisco CFIDS Foundation	965 Mission Street, Suite 425 San Francisco, CA 94103 (415) 882-9986
Southern California CFIDS Support Network	23732 Hillhurst Dr, #U-9 Laguna Niguel, CA 92677 (714) 249-6976
Utah CFIDS Association, Inc.	P.O. Box 511257, Salt Lake City, UT 84151 (801) 461-3378
Wisconsin CFS Association	P.O. Box 442, Thiensville, WI 53092 (414) 768-7560
Well Spouse Foundation	P.O. Box 801, New York, NY 10023 (212) 724-7209

Membership Form

Please, help us conquer CFIDS ✂ by becoming a member of The CFIDS Association of America today!

MEMBERSHIP BENEFITS INCLUDE:

- **Membership Packet,** including a Support Network Sheet for your area. This sheet contains the most up-to-date information on local support groups and physicians nominated to the Association's Honor Roll.

- **Subscription to** *The CFIDS Chronicle*, the largest and most comprehensive CFIDS periodical in the world.

- **Special updates** on major media, political or medical events concerning the CFIDS community.

- **Participation** in the world's largest and most active organization dedicated to conquering this disease.

The suffering inflicted by CFIDS can only be stopped through education, enlightened public policy and research — the three areas in which The CFIDS Association of America leads the nation. We want to continue the programs which have brought early and impressive progress. We want to mobilize mainstream medicine to eradicate this disease. We can only accomplish our mission by building our membership and increasing our base of support. **Please help us sustain these critical programs by joining the Association today and, if possible, by sending an additional contribution for CFIDS research, CFIDS advocacy, and/or for the Association's general operations (unrestricted).** All earmarked donations are used exclusively — dollar-for-dollar — for the specified purpose.

Annual membership dues are $30 (U.S.; $40 Canadian; $55 foreign). *PWCs may request a courtesy membership if necessary. To do so please send a letter stating reason(s) for request and enclose appropriate documents to substantiate extreme financial hardship.*

The CFIDS Association of America
MEMBERSHIP & CHARITABLE CONTRIBUTIONS FORM

Please, help us conquer CFIDS by supporting The CFIDS Association of America today!

Annual Membership Dues:

$30 (U.S.; Canadian $40; overseas $55) $_____

❑ New Member   ❑ Renewal

Charitable Contributions:

Unrestricted Donations: $_____

Earmarked Donations:

   CFIDS Research $_____

   CFIDS Advocacy $_____

TOTAL ENCLOSED: $_____

Name _____

Address _____

City _____

State _____ Zip _____

Phone _____

Method of Payment:

❑ Check or money order made payable to *The CFIDS Association of America*

❑ Mastercard or ❑ Visa

  Account No. _____

  Exp. Date _____

  Signature _____

Other Requests:

❑ I'd like to send gifts of membership in The CFIDS Association of America. Please send more details.

❑ I'd like to make a stock donation. Please have the Association's Controller contact me at:

  Phone: _____

To begin/renew your membership, mail to:
The CFIDS Association of America, Inc.
PO Box 220398 • Charlotte, NC 28222-0398
800/442-3437 • Fax: 704/365-9755

Appendix J
How to Find a Doctor

The best place to begin is with the:

CFIDS Association of America
P.O. Box 220398
Charlotte, NC 28222-0398
(800) 442-3437

I would *strongly* recommend joining this group (*See Appendix I*). They have a recommended physician's list. A physician gets on this list by being recommended by a patient with chronic fatigue. If you find a good physician sensitive to fatigue issues, recommend them for the list. The CFIDS group is in the process of updating this list.

- Call local support groups in your area (*See Appendix I*).

- Call The American Holistic Medical Association (AHMA), 4101 Lake Boone Trail, Suite 201, Raleigh, NC 27607. (919) 787-5146.
  The AHMA also has a speaker's bureau. (919) 787-5146.

- Call The American College for Advancement of Medicine. (800) 532-3688 or (714) 583-7666.

Below are several physicians/groups specializing in Chronic Fatigue Syndrome/Fibromyalgia.

Our office:

Jacob Teitelbaum, M.D.; Robert Greenfield, M.D.; Alan Weiss, M.D.

139 Old Solomons Isl. Rd., Annapolis, MD 21401, (410) 224-2222

Paul Cheney, M.D., PhD.; Charles Lapp, M.D.

10620 Park Rd. #234, Charlotte, NC 28210, (704) 542-7444

Jay Goldstein, M.D.

6200 E. Canyon Rim Rd., #110D, Anaheim Hills, CA 92807, (714) 998-2780

Byron Hyde, M.D.

Nightingale Research Foundations, Ottawa, Ontario K2A OE3, Canada

James Brodsky, M.D.

4701 Willard Ave., #224,Chevy Chase, MD 20815, (301) 652-6760

Alexander Chester, M.D.

(Specializing in nasal congestion & CFS)

3301 New Mexico Ave., NW #348, Washington, DC 20016, (202) 362-4467

Alan Gaby, M.D.

(Currently on sabbatical)

31 Walker Ave., Pikesville, MD 21208, (410) 486-5656

Jorge D. Flechas, M.D.

(uses DHEA and oxytocin)

724 5th Avenue West, Hendersonville, NC 28739, (704) 693-3015

Julian Whitaker, M.D.

Wellness Institute

4321 Birth St., Suite 100, Newport Beach, CA 92660, (714) 851-1550

Michael Rosenbaum, M.D., Murray Susser, M.D

(Authors of Solving the Puzzle of CFS*)*

Corte Madera, Santa Monica, CA, (310) 453-4424.

Leo Galland, M.D.

(Specializing in parasitic infections)

133 E. 73rd Street, New York, NY 10021, (212) 861-9000

Sigita Plioplys, M.D.; Audrius Plioplys, M.D.

(Carnitine researchers)

CFS Center, Mercy Hospital, Chicago, IL 60616, (312) 445-0123

Ruth Walkotten, D.O.

427 W. Seminole Rd., Muskegon, MI 49441, (616) 733-1989

George Mitchell, M.D.

(Clinical ecology and environmental sensitivity)

2639 Connecticut Ave, NW #C-100, Washington, DC 20008, (202) 265-4092

Richard Layton, M.D.

(Clinical ecology/allergies)

901 Dulaney Valley Rd., Towson, MD 21204, (410) 337-2707

Thomas Steinbach, M.D.

(Kutapressin research)

902 Frostwood #243, Houston, TX 77024, (713) 467-6471

177

Robert E. Pieroni, M.D., Professor Int Medicine, University of Alabama

Tuscaloosa, AL 35487, (205) 348-1287

(See Appendix K, Section 9 regarding counseling.)

Appendix K

Ordering Supplies and Services

CFIDS BUYERS CLUB (800) 366-6056

Their catalogue carries many of the nonprescription supplements you will need. Their prices are usually very competitive. All profits go to CFIDS research. I strongly recommend them.

BELMAR PHARMACY (800) 525-9473

DHEA and Oxytocin tablets are available by telephone. Your doctor calls in the prescription and your credit card number. Belmar will mail the medication to you. The Oxytocin 10 units and DHEA 50 mg each cost roughly $1/day.

TO YOUR HEALTH

11809 Nightingale Circle
Fountain Hills, AZ 85268
(800) 801-1406
Magnesium/malic acid. (Fibrocare.) Valerian/lemon balm herbal remedy for sleep. Has a resource and supply catalogue for Fibromyalgia and CFIDS.

SINUS PROBLEMS, I WOULD ORDER:

A. *Sinus Survival* book (*See Appendix L*).
B. Nasal steamer: Bearhard Industries, $40. (305) 861-2536

ANTIPARASITIC HERBAL PRESCRIPTION

Tricyclin, 2 tabs three times a day after meals for 6-8 weeks. Cost is $30 for 50 tablets. Plain Artemesia annua is less expensive and likely to be less effective.(800)782-4274

SEASONAL AFFECTIVE DISORDER (SAD)

A. Info: National Organization for SAD, P.O. Box 40133, Washington, D.C. 20016.

B. To order: "Light boxes" or visors: Bio Brite, 7315 Wisconsin Ave., Suite 1300W, Bethesda, MD 20814. (301) 961-8557, (800)621-LITE

FOOD ALLERGIES

A. Book: *How to Control your Allergies*,Forman, R. Larchmont Books, 1979. ISBN 0-915962-29-2. (Recently out of print.)

B. Ultraclear: Hypoallergenic powder food to use for elimination diets (ask for an instruction booklet when ordering). From Metagenics (800)648-5883.

BODYWORK

A. Trager—Highly recommended. Very gentle, yet very powerful. I use it for my difficult Fibromyalgia patients. Call the Trager Institute in Mill Valley, CA (415) 388-2688, Fax 388-2710. Ask for a "tutor" in your area (tutors are the teachers of Trager). If none is available, ask for a practitioner in your area.

B. Rolfing: If *deep tissue* rebalancing is desired. Powerful, but not gentle. For information and referrals call the Rolf Institute (303) 449-5903; (800) 530-8875.

COUNSELING/INNER WORK

A. Workshops with Brugh Joy, M.D., are transformational and will give you deep insight into your own inner workings. Ask for the "Foundation" workshop (12 days—includes room and board—costs about $2400). More effective than a year of regular counseling. Call (800) 448-9187 for information.

B. Look in yellow pages for Jungian psychologists/psychiatrists.

C. Association for Transpersonal Psychology. Holistic counseling. Call (415) 327-2066 for referrals in your area.

D. Ask friends and your physician. Treat the first visit as a chance to see if the "chemistry" works between you and your counselor.

Appendix L
Recommended Reading

1. *Yeast Connection and the Woman:* Wm Crook; Professional Books, Inc., 1995. Just released—an excellent book!
2. *Treatment Options in CFS—A Guide for Physicians and Patients:* Jay Goldstein; Haworth Press, 1995 (publication pending).
3. *Solving the Puzzle of CFS:* M Rosenbaum and M Susser; Life Sciences Press, 1992 (ISBN 0-943685-11-7). A good review of CFS treatments—especially of infectious problems.
4. *Safe Uses of Cortisone:* Wm Jeffries WM; Charles C. Thomas Publishing, 1981 (ISBN 0-398-04531-3). A landmark monograph on adrenal insufficiency (written for physicians).
5. *Tired or Toxic:* SA Rogers; Prestige Publishers, 1990 (ISBN 0-9618821-2-3). Extensive review of chemical sensitivity problems.
6. *The Yeast Connection:* Wm Crook; Professional Books 1994 (ISBN 0-933478-11-9). Gives an overview of problems believed to be caused by yeast overgrowth. This book has been replaced by book #1 above.
7. *How to Control Your [Food] Allergies:* R Forman; Larchmont Books 1979 (ISBN 0-915962-29-2). Diagnosis and treatment of food allergies. Out of print.
8. *The Clinical and Scientific Bases of M.E./CFS:* BM Hyde; Nightingale Research Foundation, 1992. (ISBN 0-9695662-0-4). An encyclopedic review of CFS research.

9. *The Trigger Point Manual:* JG Travell and DG Simons; Williams & Wilkins, 1983 (ISBN 0-683-8366-X). A crucial text for anyone treating myofascial [muscle] pain. Chapter 4 discusses "perpetuating factors" that also are important when treating Fibromyalgia.

10. *Curing Fatigue:* DS Bell; Rodale Press, 1993 (ISBN 0-87596-161-4). Includes good common sense approaches to fatigue.

11. *Chronic Fatigue Syndrome:* DM Dawson and TD Sabin; Little, Brown and Co., 1993 (ISBN 0-316-17748-2). Overview for physicians.

12. *The Journal of Musculoskeletal Pain:* I. Jon Russell (ed.); Haworth Press, 10 Alice Street, Binghampton, NY 13904-9981. For physicians.

13. *The Journal of Chronic Fatigue Syndrome:* N Klimas (ed.); Haworth Press, 10 Alice St., Binghampton, NY 13904-7981. For physicians.

14. *The CFIDS Chronicle:* Journal of the National CFIDS Society. Comes with a membership—if you don't belong, sign up now! See Appendix I.

15. *Sinus Survival:* Robert S. Ivker; Tarcher Press, 1991 (ISBN 0-87477-684-8). Must reading for patients with chronic sinusitis.

16. *The Canary and Chronic Fatigue:* M. Ali, IPM Press, 1994 (ISBN 1-879131-04-8). Focuses on the damage to enzyme systems by environmental stresses and nutritional/herbal/lifestyle therapeutics.

17. *CFS and The Yeast Connection:* Wm Crook, Professional Books, 1992 ISBN 0933478-20-8.

Appendix M
Jay Goldstein, M.D. Protocol

A Typical CFS/FMS New Patient Treatment Protocol

Agents, tried sequentially	Onset of action	Duration of action
1. Naphazoline HCl 0.1% gtt	2-3 seconds	3-6 hours
2. Nitroglycerin 0.04 mg SL	2-3 minutes	3-6 hours
3. Nimodipine 30 mg p.o.	20-40 minutes	4-8 hours
4. Gabapentin 100-300 mg	30 minutes	8 hours
5. Oxytocin 5-10 U IM q.d. or b.i.d. or Syntocinon 1-2 puffs t.i.d.	15 minutes or 72 hours	12-24 hours
6. Pyridostigmine 30-60 mg p.o.	30 minutes	4-6 hours
7. Hydralazine 10-25 mg p.o.	30-60 minutes	6-12 hours
8. Baclofen 10 mg	30 minutes	8 hours
9. Mexiletine 150 mg p.o.	30-45 minutes	6-8 hours
10. Tacrine 10 mg	30 minutes	4-6 hours
11. Risperidone 0.25-0.5 mg	45-60 minutes	8-12 hours
12. Pindolol 5 mg b.i.d.	15 minutes-7 days	12 hours
13. Sumatriptan 3-6 mg SQ	15-30 minutes	16 hours
14. Ranitidine 150 mg b.i.d.	1 hr-1 week	12-24 hours
15. Doxepin HCl elixir 2-20 mg q.a.m.	1 hour	Variable
16. Sertraline 25-50 mg q.a.m. or Paroxetine 10-20 mg q.a.m.	1 hour-6 weeks	1-2 days
17. Bupropion 100 mg t.i.d.	30 minutes-4 weeks	8-24 hours
18. Venlafaxine 37.5-75 mg b.i.d.	1-2 weeks	24 hours
19. Glycine powder 0.4 gm/kg/d in juice	one week	24 hours
20. Felbamate 400 mg	30 minutes	6-8 hours

I halt sequential trials when the patient is virtually asymptomatic, using other medications if tolerance should develop. These drugs are all relatively free of adverse reactions and do not appreciably interact with one another. Two selective serotonin reuptake inhibitors (SSRIs) should not be given conjointly. I prefer sertraline (Zoloft) because it does not inhibit hepatic cytochrome P450 and thus does not increase serum levels of other agents metabolized by the liver. Paroxetine, however, is less likely to cause agitation and GI side effects. SSRIs do not have as effective an analgesic effect as these other agents. A patient taking Tacrine requires regular liver function tests. Using this protocol, most patients are dramatically improved in one or two office visits.

Disclaimer Medicine in an ever-changing science. As new research and clinical experience broaden our knowledge, changes in treatment and drug therapy are required. While many suggestions for drug usage are made herein, this article is intended for educational purposes only, and the author, editor and publisher do not accept liability in the event of negative consequences incurred as a result of information presented in this article. We do not claim that this information is necessarily accurate by the rigid, scientific standard applied for medical proof, and therefore make no warranty, express or implied, with respect to the material herein contained. The physician is urged to check the product information sheet included in the package of each drug he or she plans to administer to be certain the protocol followed is not in conflict with the manufacturer's insert. When a discrepancy arises between these inserts and information in this article, the physician is encouraged to use his or her best professional judgment.

We encourage you to read Dr. Goldstein's book *(See Appendix L)* before using this protocol—J.T.

Appendix N

How to Have Your Patient's Testing Done and/or Interpreted in Our Office

Except for the stool testing, most of the testing can be done well in any lab. If, however, you would like to have us run and interpret the tests and offer our recommendations, we are happy to do so. If you choose to use our laboratory, the blood tests *must* be processed in our lab within *24 hours* of being drawn. You should have a local lab do a urinalysis. The adrenal (cortrosyn) test requires an injection, and must be done in a lab near you. The results should then be sent to us, along with the specimens for the tests you want processed in our office. Stool testing alone does not require a physician's office or lab to collect samples.

Panel 1. Contains the most important and frequently helpful tests—includes interpretation of tests.

Chem 18	Free T4	Thyroid antibodies
Magnesium	TSH	Stool O&P, also includes testing for Giardia, Cryptosporidium, Ameba, WBC, and Yeast
CBC	Serum Folate	
Manual Diff	B12	
Fe, TIBC	DHEA-S	
Ferritin	HgbA1C	Interpretation and recommendations
ESR	Food Allergy panel (10 foods)	
Total T3		Cost *$991.20*

Panel 2. Contains tests that are helpful less often, but can be important.

IgE (allergy screen)	HIV (AIDS test)	CPK
Inhalation allergies (10 airborne allergens)	Stool for C. difficile	Rheumatoid Factor
	Antinuclear antibody panel	Prolactin
RPR	(SSA, SSB, RNP, SM, DSDNA, SSDNA)	
Lymes Screen		Cost $595.00

Panel 3. Stool testing only ($250)—plus interpretation of blood tests processed in another lab with recommendations ($200)   Cost $400.00

Blood and stool test and mailing kit   Cost $15.00

Test Interpretation Only   Cost $200.00

The patient's insurance may reimburse them for most or all of the test costs. If the patient belongs to an HMO, often none of the testing is covered. If you have severe fatigue, bowel complaints, and achiness, Medicare will currently cover the cost in full. *Do not send any payment if patient has Medicare.* Please be sure to send a copy (front and back) of the patient's Medicare card.

To order a test kit which will contain forms, instructions, and specimen containers for blood and stool, please write to us. A copy of the results and our recommendations will be sent to both the patient and physician.

Send requests and $15 for each kit to:

Jacob Teitelbaum, M.D.
139 Old Solomon Island Rd.
Annapolis, MD 21401
(410) 224-2222

Appendix O

Notes

Notes

187

Index

189

190

PICTURE CREDITS*

Chapter 1: A. Masear, ©1992; Chapter 2: A. Masear, ©1995; Chapter 3: A. Masear, ©1990 ; Chapter 4: Punch, ©1989; Chapter 5: Edgar Argo, ©1993; Chapter 6: Medical Economics, ©1989; Chapter 7: Edgar Argo, ©1989; Chapter 8: Swan, ©1989; Chapter 9: Edgar Argo, ©1989; Chapter 10: North American Syndicate, ©1993; Chapter 11: King Features Syndicate, ©1990; Chapter 12: Edgar Argo, ©1992; Chapter 13: Tribune Media Services, Inc., ©1989; Chapter 14: Swan, ©1989.

*Our intention was to contact all copyright holders. In certain cases this was not possible. We invite those copyright holders to contact us so we can give them proper credit.

Order Form

YES! **Please send me** *From Fatigued to Fantastic!*

$18.95 plus $4 shipping and handling per book.

Quantity_____ x $22.95

Total $_____

_____ I've enclosed my check (payable to Jacob Teitelbaum, M.D.) for $ _____

_____ Please charge my: ___Visa ___ Mastercard

Card Number _____ Exp. Date_____

Name (as it appears on card): _____

Signature _____

Name_____

Address_____

City_____ State/Province _____

Country_____ Zip _____

Return order form to:

Jacob Teitelbaum, M.D.

139 Old Solomon Island Rd.

Annapolis, MD 21401

Order by phone:

(800) FEEL-BTR

(800) 333-5287

Or Fax your order:

(410) 224-4926

Call (410) 224-2222 for information regarding volume discounts.

Order Form

YES! **Please send me *From Fatigued to Fantastic!***

$18.95 plus $4 shipping and handling per book.   Quantity _____ x $22.95

Total $ _____

_____ I've enclosed my check (payable to Jacob Teitelbaum, M.D.) for $ _____

_____ Please charge my: ___Visa ___ Mastercard

Card Number _____ Exp. Date_____

Name (as it appears on card): _____

Signature _____

Name_____

Address_____

City_____ State/Province _____

Country_____ Zip _____

Return order form to: **Order by phone:**   **Or Fax your order:**

Jacob Teitelbaum, M.D.   (800) FEEL-BTR   (410) 224-4926

139 Old Solomon Island Rd.   (800) 333-5287

Annapolis, MD 21401

Call (410) 224-2222 for information regarding volume discounts.